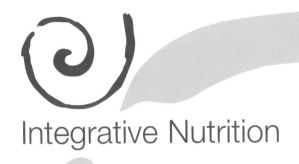

Integrative Nutrition

FAST TRACK WORKBOOK

your guide to the business of health counseling

ISBN 978-0-9773025-2-9

Published by Integrative Nutrition Publishing, Inc.
3 East 28 Street
New York, NY 10016
www.integrativenutrition.com

Printed on recycled paper.

acknowledgments

- **Joshua Rosenthal**

  for his visionary leadership, commitment and unending support of Integrative Nutrition students, alumni and staff

- **Robert Notter**

  for his dedication to Integrative Nutrition and brilliant evolution of the Fast Track program

- **Tricia Napor**

  for spearheading Integrative Nutrition Publishing with energy and focus

- **Julia Kalish, Jen Rosenblum and Erin Carden**

  for their priceless expertise and insight

- **Integrative Nutrition Staff**

  for being the most intelligent and committed group of people around

- **Integrative Nutrition Students**

  for inspiring us with their passion for learning and desire to help others

- **Alumni of Integrative Nutrition**

  for blazing the trail to a new future of health and happiness in America and the world

table of contents

introduction

Clearly, our current healthcare system is not getting people healthy. Food-related disease is the number one cause of preventable death in America. Obesity, diabetes, heart disease and certain types of cancer have all been linked to poor diet. Other health conditions, such as headaches, ADD, IBS, asthma and allergies are also rapidly increasing in America, and are beginning to spread around the world as other countries adopt America's way of life and eating habits. There are more people and children on prescriptions, medication costs are soaring, health insurance prices are higher than ever before and doctors have less time to spend with patients.

The answer to our health epidemic is not more medications and operations. The answer is prevention through diet and lifestyle. Despite the abundant advice to eat more vegetables, exercise and cut out the junk food, people are still gaining weight and getting sick. America, and the world, are in desperate need of honest health and nutrition advice that is easy and enjoyable to follow.

As a student at Integrative Nutrition, you are gaining fundamental and practical knowledge of nutrition and how to live a balanced lifestyle. This information will assist you in creating a newfound level of health and happiness in your life, and in the lives of those around you.

We encourage you to step out and use this education to be a positive influence in a world that desperately needs you. You may at first feel paralyzed and want to procrastinate getting started in this work. Learn to move beyond being a consumer of information and start to take action. Get out there, share this knowledge with other people and take a stand for what you truly believe.

If you have a passion for health and helping others, if you want a career that is fulfilling and a life that you love, now is the time to start doing this work. We are here to teach you how. This book, along with our curriculum, will take you step-by-step through how to start and run a successful business as a health counselor. You will learn to share the information you already know about health, along with the information you will learn as a student at Integrative Nutrition, with friends, family and the general public. You will become a guide, affecting many people's lives, and those people in turn will affect others. Thus we as health counselors create a ripple effect that will improve the health and happiness of people around the world.

Our mission is to dramatically improve healthcare in America. We intend to fulfill this mission with the help and hard work of committed leaders like yourself. We are incredibly grateful that you are in our school. Let the journey begin!

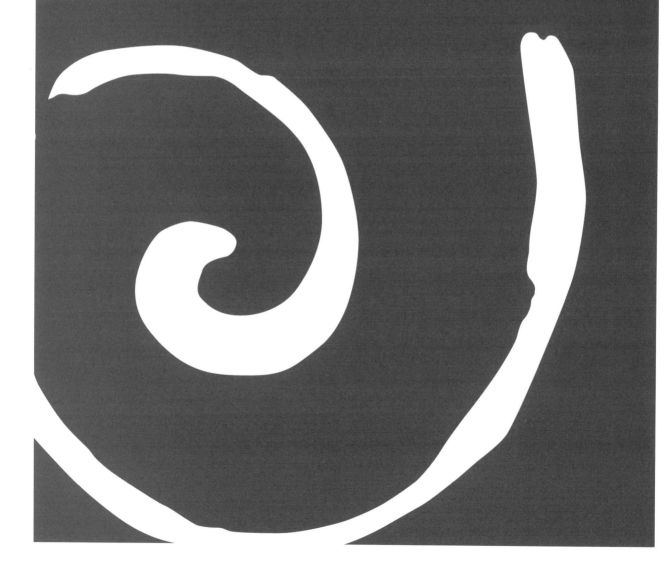

Never doubt that a small group of thoughtful,
committed citizens can change the world;
indeed, it's the only thing that ever has.

Margaret Mead,
famous anthropologist

how to use this book

follow our simple instructions

Building a business does not have to be complicated. This book, along with the curriculum taught in class, outlines our simple, time-tested process for starting your practice. Along the way you may find yourself distracted by details or tempted to overcomplicate things. Try to relax and stay focused. If you follow our simple instructions, you will experience success.

make it your own

Just as there is no right diet for everyone, there is no single business plan and structure that is best for every counselor. The information in this book reflects our years of experience helping counselors build successful businesses, but not everything in here will be exactly right for you. Use your intelligence and intuition to personalize these business strategies to work in your life.

get support

For many of you, starting your own business will be a new, challenging experience. Our community provides tremendous support to make this happen. Ask for the help you need. Use your counselor, the OEF, your buddy and your fellow students. Hold local study chapters related to business topics. Enlist your friends and family to cheer you on or to provide expert advice from their fields. Having a support team increases your chances of success.

do the exercises

Even though they may seem simple, the exercises in this book are carefully designed to walk you through the process of beginning your business. Use your pen to fill in answers and make a friendly mess of this book.

use your whole education

Don't rely only on this book to teach you how to start a business as a health counselor. The class weekends, conferences and teleclasses all provide critical information about how to be successful. This book is just one part of your curriculum. It supplements what you learn in class.

go at your own pace, but don't procrastinate

There is a lot of information in this book, and you don't have to do everything all at once. Some of these steps will be easy and fun for you. Others will be more challenging. Build your business at your own pace, but do not put it off. During the school year is when you will have the most support available. Don't miss this opportunity.

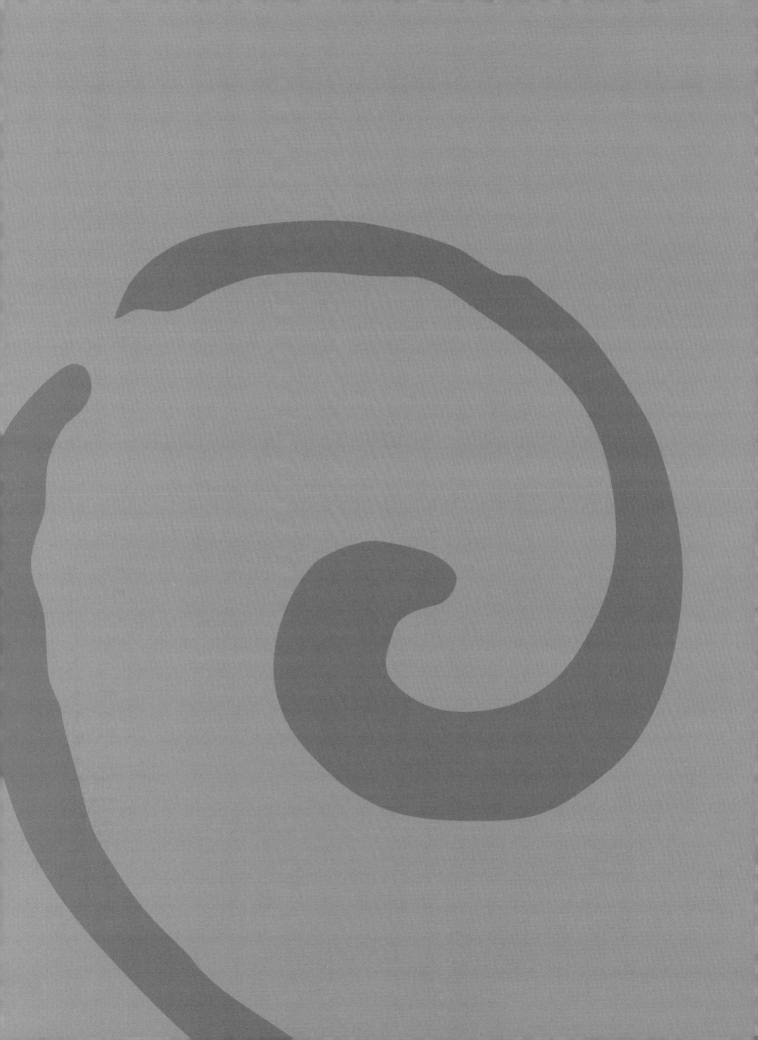

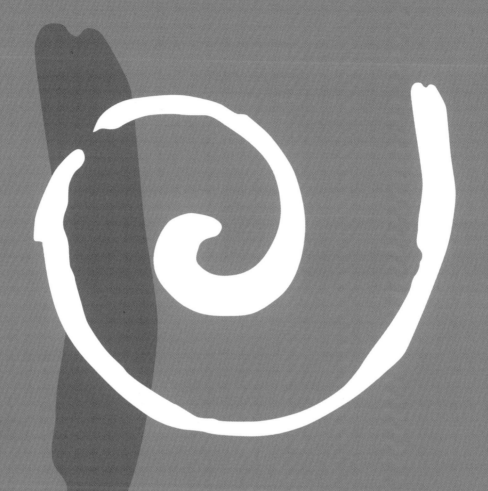

chapter one

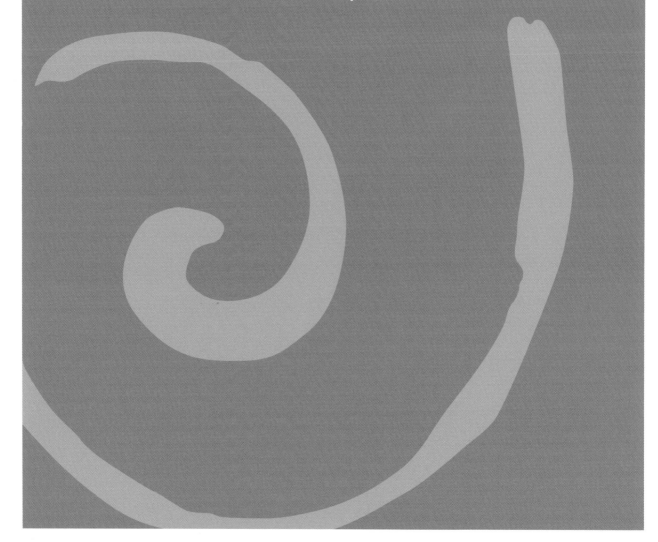

If one advances confidently in the
direction of his dreams, and endeavors
to live the life which he has imagined,
he will meet with a success unexpected
in common hours.

Henry David Thoreau

starting out as a counselor

You are on your way to becoming a certified health counselor. Congratulations! The trick to having success in this endeavor is to maintain a deep level of focus. Treat this year at Integrative Nutrition as if you were in Harvard Medical School. Work hard, pay attention, make your education a priority and follow the guidelines we set forth, and you will experience success.

Health counseling is a process in which a health counselor guides a client to reach his or her health and life goals by making step-by-step changes to diet and lifestyle. The process typically involves a six-month program. The client learns about new, healthy foods and the concept of primary foods: relationships, physical activity, career and spirituality. The health counselor works with the client to set goals to gradually incorporate improved primary and secondary foods into the client's life. Health counseling is completely focused on the client – where the client is and where he or she wants to go with his or her health and life. The health counselor acts as a guide, helping the client to gain control of and responsibility for his or her health.

career assessment

At this time, we ask that you reflect on your reasons for wanting to become a certified health counselor. Maybe it is to help other people, or maybe you want to learn how to best feed yourself. Perhaps you want to leave your current job and create a new career that you are passionate about. Whatever your reasons, please consider the following questions:

What are you doing in your current career?

_____

_____

On a scale of 1 – 10, how much do you enjoy your career?   _____

What are five things you like about your current career?

1. _____

2. _____

3. _____

4. _____

5. _____

What are five things you wish you could change about your current career?

1. _____

2. _____

3. _____

4. _____

5. _____

Please list your top five reasons for wanting to become a health counselor here:

1. _____

2. _____

3. _____

4. _____

5. _____

confidence, confidence, confidence!

The main thing that prevents our students from starting businesses as health counselors is thinking they don't know enough. This causes them to get stuck in what we call "paralization and procrastination." They put everything ahead of health counseling, saying that their lives are busy or that they have more important things to do, but underlying all of this is the belief that they will not be good enough. We do not want this to happen to you. Chances are, you are an incredibly intelligent and gifted person who has a knack for helping others. It's important for you to recognize that not everyone has these gifts.

To become a successful health counselor, you must work to increase your level of self-esteem and confidence. You are an incredibly unique person with a lot to offer the world. It is essential that you become familiar with your strengths, and that you are able to communicate them to other people. Please take a moment now to evaluate what you believe are your greatest qualities. List the top eight here:

1. _____

2. _____

3. _____

4. _____

5. _____

6. _____

7. _____

8. _____

your goals

Now we would like you to think about what you want to do with your education at Integrative Nutrition. What are your goals for building your health counseling business? How do they fit in with goals you have for other aspects of your life? This process will help clarify what you want to accomplish. In each section, please be sure to list at least one goal related to health counseling, such as the number of health histories you want to do, the number of clients you want to have, when you want to leave your current job, what kind of clients you'd like to work with or how much money you'd like to make from health counseling. Over the coming months, you will be taking consistent action to make these goals a reality.

What are three goals you have for the next week?

1. _____

2. _____

3. _____

What are three goals you have for the next month?

1. _____

2. _____

3. _____

What are three goals you have for the next six months?

1. _____

2. _____

3. _____

What are three goals you have for the next year?

1. _____

2. _____

3. _____

What are three goals you have for the next two years?

1. _____

2. _____

3. _____

What are two goals you have for the next ten years?

1. _____

2. _____

taking care of you

Starting a new career as a health counselor is exciting and rewarding. For most of you, it's an opportunity to do what you love, while simultaneously helping other people. However, starting a new business can be challenging at first. For this reason, we want you to take incredibly good care of yourself this year. In order to be a successful health counselor, you have to be healthy, happy, well rested and in balance. To support you in taking care of yourself while building your business, we will continuously do exercises, both in class and in this book, to help you stay in balance. In addition, you will have the support of your individual health counselor throughout the program to help you stay on track with self-care. We want you to be healthy and happy throughout the process, and graduate from Integrative Nutrition feeling better than ever before.

primary food

At Integrative Nutrition, we've coined the phrase "primary food." Primary food feeds us, but doesn't come on a plate. Love, hugs, touch, kisses, warmth, massage, meditation, fun, freedom, self-expression, tears, hot baths, nature, downtime, close friends and play all feed our souls and our hunger for living. These are all examples of primary foods. When our primary foods are balanced and fulfilling, our lives feed us, making what we eat secondary.

We group primary foods into four categories: healthy relationships, regular physical activity, a desired career and a spiritual practice. We invite you to look at these areas of your life from a new perspective—as a form of nutrition. This is especially important when starting this new career because your being at your best will make other people want to work with you.

Consider these four areas of your life: relationships, physical activity, career and spirituality. Write a short paragraph about each, describing any imbalances you may have in these areas and any actions you'd like to take to create more balance.

Relationships:

_____

_____

_____

_____

_____

_____

_____

Physical activity:

_____

_____

_____

_____

_____

_____

Career:

_____

_____

_____

_____

_____

_____

Spiritual practice:

_____

_____

_____

_____

_____

_____

positive thinking

Henry Ford once said, "Whether you think that you can or that you can't, you are usually right." When it comes to health counseling, this is definitely true. Believing in yourself is key to success.

Start to envision yourself as a health counselor. What does your life look like with you thriving at this work? What do your days look like? Are you a fulltime or parttime health counselor? What kind of clients do you work with? Where do you see your clients? When do you work? What do you do in your free time? Who are the key support people in your life? What health concerns have you cleared up? What else is going on in your life?

Unfortunately, we seldom have an abundance of positive thoughts in our heads. Most of us have a tendency to focus on the things in our life that are not working. That is why we at Integrative Nutrition always ask, "What is new and good?" This question breaks the habit of focusing on negative thoughts. By focusing on positive thoughts, you will attract more good into your life because what you put your attention on is what grows.

What are three things that are going well in your life now?

1. _____

2. _____

3. _____

What are three things that are going well for you so far at Integrative Nutrition?

1. _____

2. _____

3. _____

What are three things you are looking forward to about health counseling?

1. _____

2. _____

3. _____

Start to pay attention to where your mind goes most of the time. How much of your attention is on what is not going well in your life? How much attention is on what is going well?

You can incorporate positive thinking into your life in many different ways. Some simple ways are to ask people what is new and good, brag to others about what is going well with you (and then let them brag back), consciously put your mind on positive thoughts or write everything you are grateful for in a journal. Practice different ways to increase positive thinking in your life and see what works best for you. The Integrative Nutrition Journal is a great tool that incorporates food and lifestyle with gratitude and goal setting. Also, use your health counselor and your buddy for support by sharing with them what is going well in your life. Notice how you create your own reality, and that when you practice positive thinking, your world begins to look brighter.

organization

Now that you are learning to become a health counselor, it's time to start thinking of yourself as a business owner. Although this may seem overwhelming, if you take it one step at a time, you will be just fine. Use the following section to see if you have your basic necessities covered. If you answer "no" to any of these questions, you will want to take action to change your answer to "yes" as soon as possible.

basic office supplies

1. Do you have a phone?   Yes_____   No_____

If you have more than one phone number, have you chosen which one you will use for your business?   Yes_____   No_____

What is your number?   _____

Have you changed your voicemail or answering machine greeting so that it is professional? (e.g.,. "This is Jane Smith, health counselor. I cannot take your call right now, so please leave a message and I'll get back to you as soon as possible. Have a great day!")
Yes _____   No_____

2. Do you have a professional email address? (e.g. jsmith@yahoo.com)
Yes_____   No_____

If you have more than one email address, have you chosen which one you will use for your business?   Yes _____   No_____

What is your email address?   _____

If you do not have one, or you have one that is not professional, choose one here:

_____

Note: You can get free email at yahoo.com, hotmail.com or gmail.com. We suggest that you use your name if possible (e.g., janedoe@yahoo.com) rather than something less professional, such as healthmama@yahoo.com.

3. Do you have the following office supplies?

File Folders:	Yes_____	No_____
Pens:	Yes_____	No_____
Pads of Paper:	Yes_____	No_____
File Holder:	Yes_____	No_____
Calendar/Scheduling System	Yes_____	No_____
Paper Clips/Staples	Yes_____	No_____

Note: You can use your computer calendar or buy a pocket calendar.

4. Do you have a printer or access to one? Yes_____ No_____

Note: You can print at a local copy shop, Kinkos or sometimes the library.

embrace technology

Some people are afraid of technology. Are you avoiding technology? Do you know how to use your computer, email, phone and other devices? As a health counselor, your time is invaluable and using technology can certainly save you time. By learning how to work with technology, you can benefit from the fast level of service that technology provides. Also, 90% of your clients will have good technological skills and will expect you to communicate with them in this way. This is part of providing good customer service.

Here are a few fundamental things you should know how to do on your computer:
- print
- read email
- send email
- cut and paste
- save email into folders
- send attachments over email
- create Microsoft Word documents
- use CDs and discs with your computer

If you do not know how to do something from the list above, identify someone in your life who could show you. Perhaps you have a friend or family member who is good with computers.

When doing health counseling, it is imperative that you be organized. You will have appointments, follow-ups, lectures, cooking classes and events. You do not want to lose any information. There are various types of organizational systems.

file folders

Paper-filing systems can be very helpful. If you do not have filing cabinets, you can buy small, portable filing cabinets or boxes that fit file folders. You can get these kinds of supplies at Staples, Hold Everything or the Container Store. Once you have your filing cabinet, you need hanging files and file folders. To keep things neat and organized, place only one folder in each hanging file. Here are some suggested labels for your hanging files:

- Health History Forms: for blank forms. (We'll discuss what the Health History Form is in Chapter 2.)
- Health History Forms: for filled out forms. (People who did not become clients have filled these out. People who become paying clients will get their own folder and their Health History Form will go into that folder.)
- Health History Notes: for storing your ideas about what worked and what you want to improve.
- Handouts: for hard copies of all of your health counseling handouts. You will be getting a CD-ROM with all the handouts you need.)
- Clients: for information on individual clients. (Each client will have one hanging file, with a folder in each to keep that client's documents together.)
- Financial Information for copies of payment checks, receipts and any other pertinent financial information.
- Articles: for articles you collect and want to save.

computer organization

Along with your file folders and paper work, you will also want to create computer folders to save important information relevant to your business. We will be giving you CD-ROMs that will have all the forms, handouts, outlines and other documents you need to get started in your business. Once you get these, we recommend you save them onto the hard drive of your computer.

We suggest that you also create the following folders on your computer to help you stay organized with your health counseling information and documents.

- One folder called "Health Counseling" on your desktop.
- Within the "Health Counseling" folder, create folders for:
  - Forms: for soft copies of all of your health counseling forms.
  - Handouts: for soft copies of all of your health counseling handouts.
  - Classes: within this, you can create a new folder for each talk you give (e.g., Sugar Blues, Eating for Energy).
  - Newsletters: for drafts of your newsletters.
  - Marketing Ideas: for tracking business marketing ideas.

computer files or file folders

Even if you are extremely computer savvy, please know that you can not keep everything on your computer when it comes to health counseling. Your clients will be filling out Health History Forms in person and you will have papers—such as the Program Agreement—that you will want to save. So you should have an actual file folder for each client that contains their paperwork, as detailed above.

schedule organization

Some people prefer to do all their scheduling electronically, either on their computer or on a Personal Digital Assistant (PDA), such as a Palm Pilot or iPaq. Other people prefer to use an old-fashioned pocket, desk or wall calendar. Use whichever works best for you. Being organized means putting EVERYTHING into your schedule. You should put down when you plan to exercise, when you are having dinner with your family and every other little detail. Even if it is something that you are sure you won't forget, if you don't put it in your schedule, your chances of forgetting about it or double booking yourself are much higher. Your scheduling system should be foolproof. The benefit to having a pocket calendar or PDA is that you can always have it on you. Electronic scheduling systems will also set off reminders, which is great if you are a forgetful person or like to have that extra reminder.

contact organization

As you begin your health counseling business, you will meet many, many people. Some of these people will be potential clients, others will be contacts that may be able to refer clients to you or help your business in some way. You will want to keep track of important people you meet so that you can be sure to follow up with them when needed. Some people like to keep track of all their contacts via their computer, while others prefer a hard copy notepad or Rolodex. This is really a case of personal preference. Any way that works for you is great. Just make sure that you are doing something to stay organized.

One option is to keep track of your contacts by using a contact management software package such as Act! (www.act.com). With Act!, you can store contact and client information, and track any communications you have with those people.

If you do not wish to purchase a contact management software package, you can do the same kind of tracking in a low-tech kind of way. Simply use the following form to record information about people you meet. You can store these forms either in a hanging file or an online folder you create for "Contacts."

If these both feel too complicated to you at this time, you can use a Rolodex, address book or whatever works for you to keep track of your contacts. Many people collect business cards, keep them in random places and eventually lose them. Then, a few months later, they think, "I should get in touch with that woman I met who was interested in working with me. I wonder where I put her card?" You get the picture. We encourage you to organize your contact information because everyone you meet is a potential client who could lead you to many more potential clients.

contact information

Name: *the person's name and what they prefer to be called*	How you met: *e.g. friend, referral, networking event, coworker*
Home Phone: *their main contact #'s* Work Phone:	Email: *their permanent email address*
Street Address:	City, State, Zip:

Special Information:
any special details here about the person, perhaps the work they do, the name of their dog, their spouse or partner, anything that is important and that, by your remembering, would make them feel they are special to you

contact information

Name: *the person's name and what they prefer to be called*	How you met: *e.g. friend, referral, networking event, co-worker*
Home Phone: *their main contact #'s* Work Phone:	Email: *their permanent email address*
Street Address:	City, State, Zip:

Special Information:
any special details here about the person, perhaps the work they do, the name of their dog, their spouse or partner, anything that is important and that by your remembering, makes them feel they are special to you

* These forms will be on the CD-ROM you receive in class, so you can print them out and/or save them to your computer.

correspondence

Date	write down what you talked about, what you need to follow up with, and when
e.g., 12/20/05	*Initial call to set up "get to know each other" session. Scheduled for 12/22 at 7 pm in the lobby of the Marriott. Email her on 12/21 with reminder notice.*

start now

Throughout the coming months, you are going to learn a great deal of information about health and nutrition by coming to class, listening to the Visiting Teachers, reading the books, participating in the Online Education Forums (OEF) and speaking with your individual health counselor. However, it is in seeing clients while you are a student in the Professional Training Program (PTP) that you will get the most out of this education.

The current trend in America is consumerism. People are used to buying a product and then owning it. We encourage you to break this trend when it comes to your education at Integrative Nutrition. Instead of merely absorbing the information we teach and keeping it inside your brain, we want you to go out and teach others what you are learning here. Make your education an active experience.

It is through your work with clients that our curriculum will genuinely start to make sense to you. You will see how desperately in need most people are of someone to talk to about their health. By taking on clients, you will learn to become a leader and a partner in the change that is happening around health in this country. As you teach others to eat more nutritious foods and balance their lives, you will notice that you too experience growth, improved health, increased happiness and more fulfillment.

We will tell you when you are ready to start seeing clients in a six-month program. Some of you will get one client, some of you will get 20. It is required that you have at least one client before graduation. Your clients will pay you, or maybe you will barter services. Either way, it is extremely important that you start seeing clients while you are in the school because you will then have the weekend classes, your health counselor and the community of students to support you and answer any questions that may come up.

You can practice the Health History Consultation, a free initial consultation with a prospective client, while you are waiting to work with actual clients. The next chapter will explain everything you need to know about Health Histories (HHs).

Throughout the years, we have seen many students who come to class, learn all about nutrition, improve their own health and plan to do health counseling after they graduate. But this plan rarely works. These people end up putting off getting clients and never get around to it. You do not want to be one of these people. You want to use the school to help you improve your own health and then go out to help others. There is no time like the present.

I was a business analyst when I came to Integrative Nutrition, but halfway through the school year I left my job to pursue health counseling full time and teach fitness classes part time. I love being my own boss. I have a home office so I no longer have to commute. I'm making measurable differences in peoples' lives rather than feeling that I don't matter as an employee. I'm amazed at how quickly everything changed!

From the day I signed up for the program, I consistently told friends, family, colleagues and acquaintances that I was becoming a health counselor. I got a buzz going before starting to see clients in January. I was proactive and took it one step at a time, following the instructions the school gave us. I felt inspired and empowered, and I used the support from the school to take charge of my life. When I graduated in June, I had 17 paying clients!

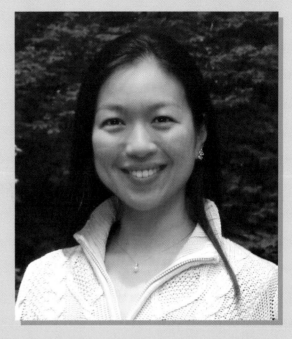

Naoko Ikeda
Harrison, NY
naoko@nourished-living.com
2006 Graduate

Public speaking has always been one of my biggest fears, but with the school's help, I actually learned to love it. The first time I led a workshop, I had trouble sleeping the night before because I was so nervous. I kept it small and invited only people I knew. For the first few minutes was uncomfortable, but by the middle of the talk I felt connected to the group and saw that they were really enjoying themselves and getting something out of it. As I continued to do more public speaking, I learned to relax more, be myself and have fun. Now my talks and workshops are so powerful because they create community and connection among my clients and prospective clients.

I've found it's really important to present myself in a professional way. Before I step outside each day, I believe I am a health counselor and move with that intention. I remind myself why I am doing this. I feel I am in demand. I'm not being pushy or asking anyone for a favor. What's amazing is that when you take care of yourself and organize your life, you get the right clients at the right time. So many people need us, so get out there and be confident!

The school provides all the outlines and materials you need, so don't reinvent the wheel. You can make it more your own whenever you are ready. At first, keep it simple and work with what you have. I got my business rolling because I didn't wait until I was perfectly ready. My price increased as my confidence and skills improved.

I love being a motivator for clients to get excited about themselves. I give them the energy to tap into their talents and live authentically. I help them find their strengths and let them shine through. I particularly enjoy helping stressed-out women prioritize their health goals. I teach them to nurture themselves, which in turn improves every aspect of their lives. As I help increase the quality of my clients' lives, I am improving the quality of my own life. I can't ask for a more fulfilling career!

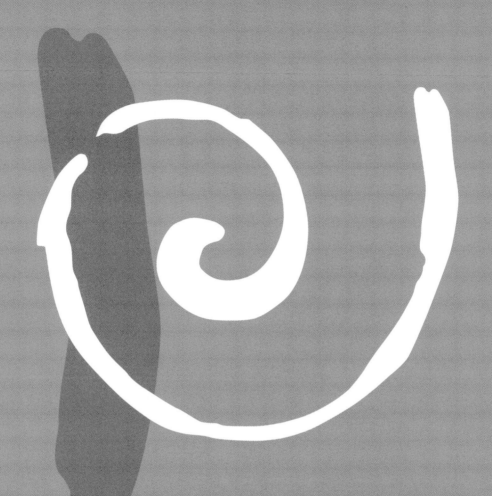

chapter two

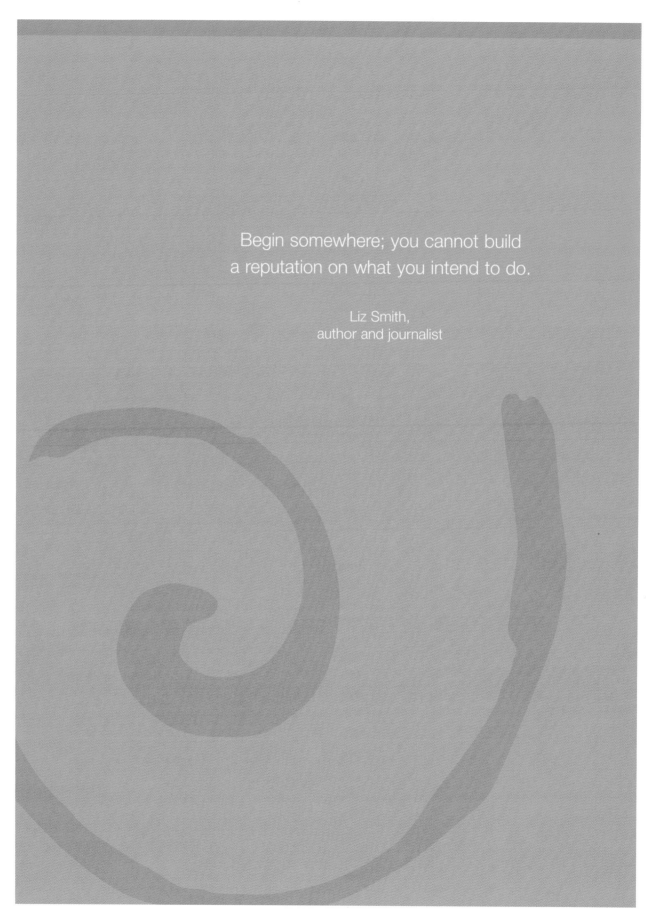

Begin somewhere; you cannot build
a reputation on what you intend to do.

Liz Smith,
author and journalist

the health history consultation

t̶he way to get a lot of clients is to do a lot of Health History consultations. A Health History is a free initial consultation that gives both you and your potential client a chance to get to know one another and determine whether or not you want to work together. The potential client gets to see what you're about—how you work and what you offer. And you get to decide whether or not the other person is someone you want to work with. Because the session is free, you are going to be more likely to have people willing to meet with you than if they had to pay for it.

the health history form

Here is the Health History Form. You want to become very familiar with this form. Take a moment now to look at all the questions. On the front are questions about the person's lifestyle and health—where they were born, what they do for a living, what their main health concern is, etc. On the back is a section about food, where the person can tell you what they ate as a child, what they ate a year ago and what they are eating now.

confidential health history

Please write or print clearly

Name:_____

Address:_____

Email address: _____How often do you check email?_____

Telephone – Work:_____ Home:_____ Cell: _____

Age:_____ Height:_____ Date of Birth:_____ Place of Birth: _____

Current weight:_____ Weight six months ago:_____ One year ago: _____

Would you like your weight to be different?_____ If so, what? _____

Relationship status:_____ Children?_____

Occupation:_____ Hours of work per week: _____

Do you sleep well? _____ Do you wake up at night? _____ What times? _____

To urinate? _____ What time do you generally get up in the morning?_____

Constipation/Diarrhea? _____ Explain:_____

What blood type are you? _____ What is your ancestry? _____

Women: Are your periods regular? _____ How many days is your flow? _____ How frequent? _____

Painful or symptomatic? _____ Please explain: _____

Do you take any supplements or medications? If so, which?_____

_____

Are there any healers, helpers or therapies with which you are involved? Please list: _____

_____

What role does exercise play in your life? _____

Do you drink coffee, smoke cigarettes, or have any major addictions? _____

What percentage of your food is home cooked? _____ Where do you get the rest from? _____

Serious illness/hospitalizations/injuries?_____

What is your chief concern? _____

Other concerns?_____

How is the health of your mother? _____

How is the health of your father? _____

confidential health history—part two
Please write or print clearly

What foods did you eat often as a child?

Breakfast	Lunch	Dinner	Snacks	Liquids
_____	_____	_____	_____	_____
_____	_____	_____	_____	_____
_____	_____	_____	_____	_____
_____	_____	_____	_____	_____
_____	_____	_____	_____	_____

What about one year ago?

Breakfast	Lunch	Dinner	Snacks	Liquids
_____	_____	_____	_____	_____
_____	_____	_____	_____	_____
_____	_____	_____	_____	_____
_____	_____	_____	_____	_____
_____	_____	_____	_____	_____

What's your food like these days?

Breakfast	Lunch	Dinner	Snacks	Liquids
_____	_____	_____	_____	_____
_____	_____	_____	_____	_____
_____	_____	_____	_____	_____
_____	_____	_____	_____	_____
_____	_____	_____	_____	_____

the health history consultation

We'll discuss later in this chapter how to find and invite people to come to your free initial Health History Consultation. But first, let's review what will happen before, during and after the consultation.

before the health history consultation

- Decide where you are going to hold the consultation:
    - at home
    - at an office
    - on the phone
    - in a hotel lobby
    - in a tea or coffee shop
- Send a reminder email a day or two before your appointment. In this email, give directions for where to meet you, and let the person know you look forward to seeing them. If the person does not regularly use email, you can call instead.
- Pick out an outfit that is professional, yet comfortable.
- Make sure you have a blank Health History Form, a pen and a clipboard to write on.
- Center yourself by quieting your mind right before the meeting.

beginning the health history consultation

- When you greet the person, give them a warm welcome. Show them you are happy to see them. Acknowledge the potential client's presence and thank them for taking the time to talk with you.
- Connect by touch—shaking hands or hugging if appropriate.
- Give the person the Health History Form to fill out on a clipboard or something that makes it easy to write on. It is best to have them fill out the form at the beginning of the session while they are with you. Filling out the form can be an emotional process, so it is good that you are there to provide support and address whatever comes up. If you prefer, you can have them fill out the form ahead of time and bring it with them to your session. This may be a better option if you know you have a limited amount of time.
- Offer the person some water or tea and get it while they are filling out the form.
- If the session is over the phone, have a blank form in front of you before the call begins. Then you can ask the questions and fill in the answers as you go through the form. If you prefer, you can email the form ahead of time and have the person fill it out and email it back to you. But again, we recommend doing it together in case anything emotional comes up.
- Once you have the completed form in front of you, you can begin the conversation. Here are some sample questions you might ask to get the conversation started:
    "So, how was filling out this from for you?"
    "What's new and good in your life?"
    "How do you feel about coming to a Health History Consultation?"

during the health history consultation

- Use the form to guide you. Go through the form in order. Ask questions based on what the person wrote on the sheet. Let them talk about everything, especially their main health concern. The form is meant to stimulate conversation. You may find that your potential client wants to talk more about one part of the form and less about another. That's OK—go where the client wants to go.

- Go over easy information first. Where they live, where they are from, how old they are, etc. You can ask questions such as, "How does it feel being 36?" or "How was it growing up in Nebraska?" or "Do you like living in New York City?"

- Listen, connect and take notes. The more you listen, the more the person will open up. Connecting with the person will create trust. And if you take notes, the person will feel important. However, avoid taking too many notes. You don't want to have your head in your paper the whole time.

- Breathe. Notice how much you like talking to and listening to this person. Empty your mind of everything that you have to do or anyplace you need to go. Stay present. Trust yourself.

- When you get to the more complex subjects, such as weight, relationships, career and sleep, read between the lines and ask questions that draw the person out. For example, if the person wrote that they want their weight to be different, you can ask, "Do you want to look slimmer, feel lighter or both?" A good question to ask if you see they spend many hours working is, "I see that you work about 45 hours each week. Does that feel like a lot to you, or does it feel like you have a good balance of work, rest and play?" If they wrote that they don't sleep well and wake up a lot during the night, you can ask "Why do you think that is?"

- People are not used to talking about their digestion in regular conversation, so you may find resistance around getting people to open up about constipation or diarrhea. It may be helpful to say something like, "Most people suffer from some kind of digestive problem. I see it all the time and talking about digestion is one of the key elements to figuring out what foods are best for you." Or share something about yourself such as, "I used to have terrible constipation, but since I changed my diet, it's cleared up, which I'm thrilled about."

- If possible, make the person laugh. If you can get someone to laugh in your office, that is a huge step forward. Most people take healthcare so seriously. Having fun with the person will make them feel comfortable and lighten the mood.

- Do not give advice during the Health History. We can not stress this point enough. Let the person do the majority of the talking. Ask questions to take them deeper into what they are talking about. In the Health History, you are simply gathering information and talking about your program. Once someone becomes your client, then you can start giving advice.

- Share how you relate to the person's issues. When someone knows that you are human too, and you have worked through your own health issues, they will feel closer to you. However, be careful to not talk about yourself too much. Mention some health conditions or health concerns that you have cleared up either once or twice throughout the Health History.

- Remember and write down key points to bring up later in the conversation. If the person shared earlier that they take allergy medication, you can say, "When I am ready to start seeing clients, I can work with you to help you understand what is going on with your allergies."
- Notice if there are any areas of the form left blank. It could be that the person did not list something because they are avoiding it. Use your judgment. You may want to say, "I notice that you did not write anything down for this question. Why is that?"
- Restate and paraphrase what the person shares with you. This shows you understand what is being communicated to you and gives the person the opportunity to clarify anything that is unclear. When the person says something, you can say, "So what you are saying is…" or "What I'm hearing you say is…"
- Briefly explain the concept of primary and secondary foods. It will be helpful for the person if you talk about the importance of both what we eat and our lifestyle, how if we are not happy or fulfilled in one aspect of our life, such as relationship or career, we will not be healthy no matter what we eat. Remember to avoid giving them any advice. Simply introduce the concept.
- Do not avoid silence. Let the person speak and when they are done speaking, you do not have to start speaking right away. Sometimes if you allow silence, the person will take this as permission to go even further with their thoughts. Real healing can occur here. Even if the silence feels awkward to you, it's okay to experiment with allowing it.
- At the end of the Health History, after you've gone over what the person is eating, ask, "What are three things you know you could be doing for your health that you are not currently doing?" Then write those down. You will use them in your closing.

ending the health history consultation

- Tell the person that you've really enjoyed getting to know them better and mention one specific thing that you liked about the session.
- Ask them, "How was that for you?" and "What was something you found valuable in our session?"
- Restate some of the health concerns the person mentioned and the three things they know they could be doing for their health. For example, you can say, "I know that your main concerns at this time are losing weight and having increased energy. It's great that you know eating less and working out more will help you with these goals. However, I find that most people know what they should be doing for their health, but they have difficulty actually doing it. If we were working together, I would be here to support you and hold you accountable."
- Explain how your six-month program works. Let the person know that you would meet twice a month for an hour, and that these sessions would be similar to the Health History. You would discuss what is going with their health, and at the end of each session you would provide them with recommendations to work on before the next session. Also let them know about the other benefits: monthly seminars or cooking classes; a health food store tour; and a variety of books, CDs and other items.

- Ask them, "Would you be interested in working with me when I am ready to see clients?"
- If they say yes, you can say something like, "Great! I will follow up with you when I am ready in about two months. What is the best way to get in touch with you?" (It is important to take control of the process. You must contact them and follow up once you are ready to start seeing clients. Do not wait for them to contact you.)
- Bonus Step: Ask them. "Do you know anyone else who you think may be interested in doing a Health History with me?" If they do, get that person's contact information.
- We'll talk more in Chapter 5 "Closing the Deal" about how to end the Health History Consultation once you are ready to see clients!

after the health history consultation

- Follow up with the potential client via email or phone. Appreciate them and mention something personal to make them feel special. Let them know you will keep them updated on when you are ready to start seeing clients.
- Keep a log of all your Health Histories in one place. You may want to create an Excel spreadsheet or use a piece of paper from your Health History folder. A suggested template is at the end of this chapter.
- Reflect on your session. What worked? What didn't work? Take notes for yourself and keep them in the binder, folder or notebook where you keep all your Health History information. Take a moment to realize that you are an amazing work in progress. Your counseling skills will only improve with time.

listening

As mentioned earlier, you should do very little talking during the Health History. People love to talk about themselves, especially with someone who is a good listener. Most health professionals today have very limited time to speak with their clients or answer questions. When people come to you, it will be a much-needed breath of fresh air. They will be thrilled to have the space to speak about what is going on with their health and their life. By simply speaking and being listened to, the people who come to you for Health Histories will make connections around their health that they would not make if it were not for your presence.

What are five things that you already do that make you a good listener?

1. _____

2. _____

3. _____

4. _____

5. _____

listening

Most people live in their heads, thinking about what they have to do tomorrow, what happened yesterday or an hour ago, pretty much anything except the present moment. Because we are all living in our own heads, we are rarely listening to what other people are saying. Likewise, it is rare that someone actually listens to us without interruption or judgment. When done well, listening delivers tremendous benefits.

As a health counselor, you are offering anyone who comes to you for a health history the priceless opportunity of being listened to. The stronger your listening skills, the better a health counselor you will be. In order to listen well, put all the thoughts about yourself out of your head. Focus on the person you are listening to. This will greatly improve the quality of your communication. Listening is an art that fosters understanding, affirmation, relatedness and appreciation.

Tips for listening well, both on the phone and in person:

- Remain curious and ask pertinent questions that bring the person deeper into what they are talking about.

- Summarize what they say to determine if you accurately understanding the speaker.

- If in person, keep strong eye contact. If on the phone, it's good to say things or make noises to let them know you are listening and comprehending what they are saying.

- Try to sit in one place. Avoid moving around.

- Learn to be comfortable with silence and being quiet. Don't talk in awkward silences; sometimes this is when the client reveals the most important information.

- Listen with your whole body: ears to hear the message, eyes to read body language (in person), the mind to visualize the person speaking (phone), intuition to determine what the speaker is actually saying.

- Meet in an environment conducive to listening. Avoid coffee or tea shops with loud music, tables that are very close together, or outside parks with a lot of children.

Things to avoid when listening:

- Looking at your watch or around the room as opposed to focusing on the speaker's face.

- Multitasking. In person—writing, cleaning, looking for something, cooking. Over the telephone—opening mail, reading email, filing, and playing with hair or a pencil.

- Constantly interrupting. This makes the speaker feel that what he or she has to say is not important.

- Finishing the other person's sentences.

inviting people to a health history consultation

Coming to a Health History Consultation with you is a great opportunity for anybody. It's important for you to know your worth when extending invitations. What you are offering is free, but it is incredibly valuable. Even if the person doesn't express interest in signing up for your program, simply talking about their health with you for an hour will be extremely beneficial.

Even though you may not be ready to see clients yet, it is necessary that you start doing Health History Consultations now to get familiar with the process. It's best to do at least one or two a week. The first ten Health History Consultations you do will be the most difficult. After that, they are simple. So get the first ten out of the way as soon as possible. Practicing Health Histories will build your confidence and you will find your own unique style and become more comfortable with the process. Also, as you do Health History Consultations the word will begin to spread about the new work you are doing. If you do a lot of Health History Consultations now, you will have people waiting to sign up for your six-month program when you are ready to start seeing clients.

Please take a moment now to make a list of five people who you know with whom you could do a Health History Consultation. In the beginning, you may feel more inclined to ask family and coworkers, but we find that working with family members and coworkers can get complicated. Friends or acquaintances usually make better clients.

1. _____

2. _____

3. _____

4. _____

5. _____

In addition to this list, part of being a health counselor is talking to strangers about what you do. Potential clients are everywhere: at the health food store, the gym, yoga class, the bookstore, church, temple, on the bus, at the bank, EVERYWHERE! List five places that you know of where you think you could find someone who would want to do a Health History Consultation with you.

1. _____

2. _____

3. _____

4. _____

5. _____

You may be very comfortable talking to strangers, or you may not. If you don't, that's okay. You will learn. Start off slowly and build up your muscle for starting conversations with people.

communicating with potential clients

Once you are familiar with the Health History Form and you have a list of people to contact, you are ready to start inviting people for a free consultation. Begin by contacting everyone on the first list above. You can then make plans to go to the places on the second list and talk to people.

Depending on how prepared and confident you are at this time, you may invite people for a Health History now, or maybe you will start building relationships, letting them know what you are up to, and actually invite them for a Health History later. Of course, we encourage you to start now. There is no time like the present! At this point in time you are not looking to actually get clients enrolled in a paid program; your goal is simply to do Health History Consultations.

In general, we recommend that you tell everyone you know what you are doing and invite them to come for a free Health History. Tell your friends, colleagues, acquaintances—everyone.

You can send out a professional, warm email to all of your contacts, inviting them to a Health History. You can also send a casual email out to your close friends seeing if they are interested, or if they know someone who might be interested in doing a Health History Consultation with you. We have included sample emails for you in the next section of this chapter.

If someone asks you what a Health History is, you can say, "We will spend about an hour going through your Health History and discuss what you eat, your lifestyle and any goals for your health. We will also get a sense of how it would be to work together. How does that sound?"

Share how excited you are and how much your life has improved since changing your diet and lifestyle. You can give them an example of a health concern that you have cleared up or something that is going really well with you as a result of getting involved with the school and health counseling. This will inspire them to want to have more of what you have!

Here are some examples of what to say when inviting people for a Health History Consultation:

• "I am taking this course at a nutrition school in New York City and I have a homework assignment to do some Health History Consultations. Would you be interested in sitting down with me for an hour while we discuss your health?"

• "Do you think you have an hour sometime this week to sit down with me and talk about your health? We can look at how what you are eating is affecting your health."

• "Have you ever thought about how what you eat affects your health? I'd be happy to talk with you about it further in a free consultation."

• "I have some exciting news. I am in school to become a certified health counselor. I'd love to show you what I'm learning. Would you like to sit down with me and discuss what is happening in your life and with your health?"

• "I am a student at Integrative Nutrition in New York City, studying to be a certified health counselor. I am learning about how food, diet and lifestyle have a tremendous impact on our overall health, happiness and well-being. Not only am I learning to improve my life, I am being very carefully and skillfully instructed on how to see clients and help them to reach their health goals and to feel and look better."

- Ask the person, "I'm curious, what is one area of your health you would like to improve?" or "What is your main health concern?" After they respond, you can say something like, "Actually, part of my course requirements and homework are to do free health consultations with other people. I'd be happy to sit down with you and have a conversation about your health goals. Would you be interested in doing a Health History Consultation with me?"

If inviting a person to do a Health History is scary, you can practice telling people that you are studying to be a health counselor. From there, they will most likely ask what a health counselor is or what you are studying in school. You can tell them, "I help people discover how what they eat affects their health" or "I work with people to help them improve their diet and lifestyle." Listen to how they respond and if it is positive, you can say, "Would you be interested in doing a free consultation with me?" Another approach to take would be to talk to people about something you learned in class. For example, if you are in a social setting you can say: "Last weekend in class I heard from the head of nutrition at Harvard and he said…" From there, they may ask more about what you are studying. If they sound interested, you can invite them for a Health History.

Be yourself. Say whatever is true for you. With time and practice, you will find your personal style and language.

sample email 1

Please adapt to fit your own unique style.

Dear (name),

I have some exciting news! I am beginning a new business as a health counselor, in which I will be working with people on how to improve their diet and lifestyle. My business is in the early stages and I am currently offering free health consultations. I was wondering if you would be interested in having a session with me. We would get together for an hour and talk about your health, past and present. Please let me know when is a good time for you to get together. Monday and Tuesday evenings, after 6pm, are usually best for me. Also, if you know anyone else who you think would benefit from talking with me about their health, feel free to forward them my contact information.

I look forward to hearing from you

Regards,
Counselor Name

sample email 2

Please adapt to fit your own unique style.

Hello, (name)!

I hope you are well, and that (personal note, e.g., "your husband Tom is doing well at his new job"). I am writing because I'm very excited to share something new and good that is happening in my life. I recently decided to begin training in a new career path, and I enrolled at the Institute for Integrative Nutrition in New York City. I am learning to become a certified health counselor. As you know, I have always had an interest in health (or nutrition or healing) and have enjoyed sharing this knowledge with my friends, colleagues and family. I decided that I wanted to increase this knowledge and learn, in a formal training program, how to live a better life through eating well and taking care of myself. Not only am I learning how to take care of me, I am also receiving very detailed and careful instruction on how to counsel others around food and lifestyle choices. It's an exciting time!

Part of my course requirements and homework are to do free health consultations with other people. I'd like to invite you to do a session with me. I'd be happy to have the opportunity to support you in living an even happier, healthier life. In this consultation, we will spend about an hour going through your Health History and your goals for your health. We will also get a sense of how it would be to work together once I am able to start seeing clients.

I'd appreciate an opportunity to share this session with you, and allow you to have time to talk about your health and life. The session is free and confidential and we can meet wherever it's convenient for you.

Please let me know what your schedule is like in the coming 1-2 weeks, and when you might have time to talk. I will contact you again on (5 days later) to follow up if we don't have a chance to speak before then.

I look forward to hearing from you, and I hope you have a great day.

Regards,
Counselor Name

scheduling health history consultations

Read the next sentence very carefully. If someone expresses interest in doing a Health History with you, schedule it on the spot! Set the exact time and tell them where the Health History will be. You can say, "Great! I am free on Tuesday and Thursday nights and Sunday afternoons. Would any of those times work for you?" Or you might say something like, "I would love to set up a free consultation with you. My schedule can get full very quickly, so is it okay if we schedule it now? What days and times work best for you next week?" This means that you should start to carry a planner with you at all times, because you never know when you are going to meet potential clients. You also want to make sure you get the person's phone number and email. Let them know you will email them the details of when and where to meet you. Within 24 hours, email them the address, your phone number and the date and time of your appointment. You will also send them a reminder about your appointment 24 hours beforehand.

If you skip this crucial step of immediately scheduling appointments, you will lose out on potential clients. Believe us – people are not going to knock down your door to schedule a Health History with you. This is not because they don't want to work with you. This is because they are busy and they do not prioritize their health. They put their jobs, relationships and a million other things ahead of their own well-being. They need you to be the advocate for the importance of their health. You can do this for them by being assertive in scheduling the initial consultation. You are not doing anyone any favors by playing small or being shy.

If you don't have your schedule, or it is not an appropriate situation in which to schedule the Health History, get the person's contact information and be in touch within 24 hours to set up the appointment.

frequently asked questions and suggested answers

Sometimes, when scheduling a Health History or during the actual Health History, people will ask you questions you may or may not have the answers to. In these situations, it is best to answer the question honestly. If you don't know the answer, you can say, "That's a great question, I will look into it and get back to you."

Also, you can practice ahead of time by anticipating potential questions and deciding on the best responses. You can also write down questions people ask you during the Health History, and keep a list of them for future reference.

Here are a few of the questions you may get and some suggested replies:

• What is a Health History?
"During a typical consultation, we will spend about an hour going through your Health History and your goals for your health, and what you've always imagined for your life. We will also get a sense of how it would be to work together. How does that sound?"

- What is a health counselor?

"A health counselor guides you to reach your health and life goals by making step-by-step changes to your food and lifestyle, at a pace that's comfortable for you."

If people who are not clients ask you for advice, try not to give them recommendations. Instead, say: "I just started my training program, and for now I'm not giving recommendations. That is a great question though, and those concerns you mentioned are the types of things we would cover together if you were to become my client."

- Are you really qualified to see people before you finish your training?

"It is very common that other professionals like lawyers and psychologists begin to see clients/patients before the end of their training, just like I do as a health counselor. This coming June, I will be fully certified by the American Association of Drugless Practitioners."

- What about confidentiality?

"Like any other health professional, I keep everything clients share with me strictly confidential."

- How does the program work?

"I will be working with clients in six-month health counseling programs. During the six months, I will meet my clients individually twice a month and help them to reach their goals for their life and their health. Together, we will look at their current diet and lifestyle and customize a plan for how to upgrade their food and other aspects of their life. I will also offer cooking classes, a health food store tour, books and CDs on health-related topics and other fun ideas to help improve their health. Right now I am offering free initial consultations. I will begin to see clients in a few months."

- Why is it six months?

"Studies show that if you do something for six months, it is likely to become a long-term habit. My goal is that after six months of working together with a client, they will have a deep understanding of the foods and lifestyle that work best for them. I want them to take what they learn through working with me and use it for the rest of their life."

keeping track of clients

As you begin inviting people to Health History Consultations and lining up potential future clients, you will need a way to keep track of it all. At a minimum, we recommend that you keep track of the person's name, their email and phone numbers, the date of their Health History Consultation, and any relevant notes that you will want to remember. You will especially want to remember whether or not they are a potential client for you once you are ready to start seeing clients. We've included a sample Health History Tracking Form at the end of this chapter—feel free to make Xerox copies of it, or recreate it on your computer. You can also edit it in any way that makes sense to you. The important thing is that you keep track.

health history tracking form

Name	Phone	Email	Date of HH	Potential Client?	Follow-Up Notes

health history excitement

We understand that the idea of doing a Health History with someone is a new concept for you. You probably have a myriad of different thoughts and emotions about this, from fear to excitement and nervousness.

List three things that you are nervous about:

1. _____

2. _____

3. _____

You can use your counselor, the OEF (Online Education Forums) and your fellow students to help you work through anything that you are nervous about. Remember to feel the fear and do it anyway!

We ask that instead of focusing on what is scary, you focus your attention on your excitement. In fact, all nervousness usually comes out of excitement. Allow yourself to be happily energized about this new adventure you are beginning.

List three things that are exciting regarding doing Health Histories:

1. _____

2. _____

3. _____

Also, remember to have fun!

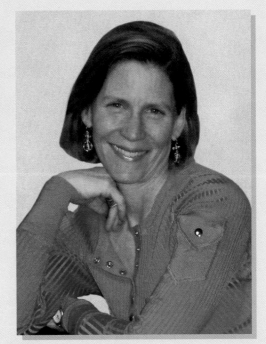

I worked in advertising in New York City for 15 years before I came to Integrative Nutrition. I enjoyed what I was doing, but I was exhausted from working 15-hour days, and I wanted to be home with my kids. Food was always important to me, as was feeding my kids really well. As soon as I entered the doors of Integrative Nutrition, I knew I wanted to make a career out of health counseling. My goal from day one was to make my tuition investment back by the time I finished the program. It was a great motivator for me to get my business started.

The biggest step I took to build my practice while in school was affiliating with an integrative medical practice. I met one of the doctors through a friend of a friend, and invited her to have lunch with me. I asked her to seriously consider having me in the office. I explained to her that it was a win/win proposition. She would make money by renting space to me, and it would give her the credibility of having a truly integrated practice by adding a nutrition expert to her staff. She agreed! I graduated the program with 15 clients, and about half of them were referrals from the doctors there.

Frances Murchison
Lake Forest, IL
frances@mindfullyfed.com
2003 Graduate

I moved to Chicago shortly after graduation and found myself having to start all over again. I didn't know a soul, so I decided I would make some friends with people who had lived in the area for a long time and offer free cooking classes to their contact lists. I met one friend who was willing to provide me with the names and addresses of 50 people in the area. I sent them all hard-copy invitations to a cooking class, and about 30 people accepted. Five people signed up for my program. I continued setting up paid cooking class series and other group events, and within six months I had 15 clients!

I recommend that you make it a point to tell at least three people each day what you're doing. The more people you tell, the more you will believe in yourself and get comfortable in your new role as a health counselor. Another tip is to stick to the policy of having clients pay up-front. When I first started, I bent over backwards to accommodate people because I was afraid they would say no to my program. The more I set boundaries and raised my rates, the more people wanted my service.

I learned everything I know about building a business at Integrative Nutrition. I had always dreamed of being an entrepreneur, but I was scared to death, so stayed in my corporate job. For the first time in my life, I feel like I am doing what I am meant to be doing. I have finally figured out how to take my wisdom and experience and offer it back to the world.

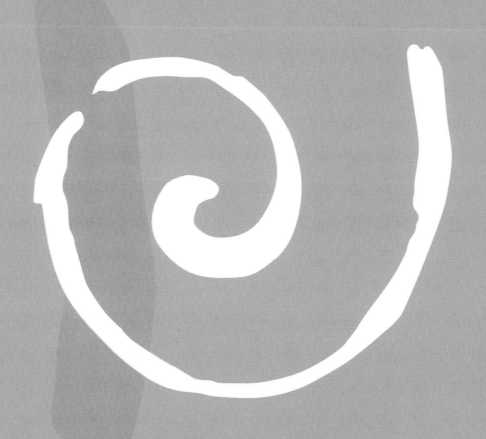

chapter three

Pleasure in the job puts perfection in the work.

Aristotle

setting up your business

Once you've completed several Health Histories and have a clear idea of what health counseling is, you are ready to set up your business. Having a legitimate business will help you look and feel more professional. It is also important to officially start your own business so that you will be in adherence with any business laws in your state.

For many of you, running your own business may be a lifelong dream—the step you need to free yourself from working for others, and accomplish your own goals. In this chapter, we'll review some basic steps for getting your business up and running, including creating your office, determining your business name and your title, picking a legal structure, how to register, creating a website, setting up bank accounts, accepting credit cards and managing finances.

This book cannot substitute for the legal, financial and other professional advice required when establishing or expanding a business. While every effort has been made to ensure that the information included in this book is accurate, we urge you to consult with your state's appropriate agencies and work with a qualified professional before actually proceeding to establish a business.

forms

All of the forms you will need to run your health counseling business are included in the CD-ROMs you will receive over the course of the school year. When you get each CD-ROM, you should save it to your computer and spend some time reviewing everything that is on it. You can also customize the forms as you see fit, adding your logo, name or contact information.

There are certain forms on the CD-ROMs that you may want to print out and have on hand, such as the Health History Form, Program Agreement and any other forms that you use on a regular basis. One suggestion is to have client folders ready to go, each containing a blank Health History Form, Program Agreement, Client Progress Form and Giveaway Checklist. This way when you have a Health History you just grab one of the folders, rather than printing out and organizing all the paperwork each time.

You may want to staple the Client Progress Form to the left side of the folder and the Giveaway Checklist to the right side. After each session, you can easily mark down how the session went and what you gave to your client. If you can find a way that works for you to organize all your forms and paperwork, it will save you a lot of time and stress in the future.

office set-up

When you first begin health counseling, it's completely okay for you to not have an office. You can meet your clients in a coffee shop, library, bookstore, their home, your home or a hotel lobby. There will be advantages and disadvantages to consider with each. You will want to meet your clients in a comfortable setting where you can speak about personal topics.

Eventually you will want to get office space. An office space will allow you to stay in one place to see your clients, and guarantee that you have the exact environment you want. You may rent an office or create one in your home.

If you choose to rent an office, consider renting in a massage therapy practice, a wellness center or a therapist's office, with other health professionals who might refer clients to you. You can also rent space from community centers, YMCAs and churches at reasonable rates. Some health counselors get together in groups of two to four and rent a single office, splitting the rent to make it more affordable.

If you use your home as your office, it's helpful to pick an area of your house where you will see clients. It may be at your kitchen table or on your couch. Perhaps you have a room that you can turn into your office. If you don't have an area that works, think about purchasing Japanese screens and sectioning off a small area of your home where you can fit two chairs and a small table.

You'll need at least two comfortable chairs in your office. You'll also need a clock, strategically placed so that you can easily view it during your sessions and keep track of time. You may also want to have attractive decorations, a hot pot for making tea, a CD player to play relaxing music and a bookshelf to display all of your books. It's up to you—be yourself!

You will also need office space to do all of your paperwork and correspondence. This may or may not be the same place where you see your clients. Regardless, there are certain things you can have set up in your "working" office to help you be organized and ready to go:

- clock
- printer
- computer
- fax machine
- phone with headset
- corkboard for the wall
- file cabinets—at least one
- space to store your client giveaways
- comfortable, ergonomically correct desk and chair
- pens, pencils, computer printer paper, notebooks, binders, etc.

If your working office is different from the place you see clients, you will also need a convenient way to transport materials, such as forms, giveaways and clipboards, to your client sessions. Set aside one bag or backpack to take to your client sessions that is stocked with everything you need and keep it in a convenient place so that you can grab it when you go out to see clients.

creating a business name

There is no "one-size-fits-all" formula for picking a fantastic business name. There are a few things to consider—such as the kind of business you do, your target market and your unique style or personality. Here are a few criteria that your business name should meet:

- is distinctive
- is memorable
- suggests the services you offer
- is easily spelled and pronounced

The options for your business name are endless. You can use your first or last name as part of your business name, such as Jane Smith Health or Health with Jane. Or, you can pick a powerful name that conveys what your business is about without including your name. Words such as "health," "nurturing" and "wellness" are popular among our students and graduates.

Write six possible business names here:

1. _____

2. _____

3. _____

4. _____

5. _____

6. _____

Which of these do you think is the strongest and most representative of what you do? If you are not sure, you can ask your friends, family, fellow students and health counselor what they think. We suggest you give yourself a few weeks before finalizing your decision and registering your business name.

Make sure that someone else does not already have the rights to use the name you have chosen. Here are three steps you can take in conducting a name search:

- A quick and easy place to start is with an online search engine, such as Google. When you google the name you like, what else comes up? Is there clearly another business with this name?

- Go to www.networksolutions.com and type in the name you want to use. If another company has reserved a domain name that contains the business name you want, you probably won't be able to use it because the domain name qualifies as a trademark if the website is used commercially.

- Get in touch with your county clerk's office. There you can check a list of all the assumed business names in the country. In some states, you can also check with the state corporation commission to view a database of all business names.

If someone else is using the business name you want to use, you shouldn't use it.

You might also want to check that your business name can be used as a website address, also called domain name or URL. These days, most successful businesses have websites. Having your website match your business name allows potential clients to find you quickly and easily. For example, if your business name is "Health with Jane," you might want to use www.healthwithjane.com as your domain name. It can be difficult to find a domain name that is not already taken. To find out if the one you want is available, go to www.networksolutions.com. If the .com of your company name is taken, you can always use .net or .tv.

More information is provided below about how to connect your domain name with your free student website provided by Integrative Nutrition.

your title

We think that the term "health counselor" is the most accurate description of what our students and graduates practice with their clients. Your Integrative Nutrition diploma will say that you are a Certified Health Counselor. However, you do not have to use this title. Some graduates choose to call themselves holistic health counselors, health coaches or lifestyle coaches. It's up to you. Be careful, however, about picking titles that require certain qualifications that you do not have. For example, you cannot call yourself a registered dietician in any of the states unless you are registered with the American Dietetic Association. Also, if you decide to use the term "coach," you cannot call yourself certified. Most states also have strict guidelines on who can use the term "nutritionist."

determining your business structure
and registering your business

Once you choose your business name and title, you can register your business so that you are in adherence with state or local regulations in your area. The process of registering your company with your state and local governments will vary depending on the business entity type. This section describes the most common forms of business entities. All this business information may seem overwhelming at this time. Breathe. And read each section slowly and carefully. We will talk about this more in class to provide any additional support. We included it here to give you a clear picture of what your options are.

sole proprietorships

Most new businesses, and most students at Integrative Nutrition, start as sole proprietorships because it is the easiest, cheapest and quickest way to create a business. In fact, about 70% of small businesses are sole proprietorships. This type of business is an option if you are going to be the only person who owns the business. If you have co-owners or partners, sole proprietorships are not allowed, unless your partner is your spouse.

A sole proprietorship is a business that is owned by one individual, and is unincorporated. It is the simplest form of business organization to start and maintain. In a sole proprietorship the business and its owner are one and the same. The business has no existence apart from you, the owner. Therefore, you are solely responsible for your business. Its liabilities are your personal liabilities. Your business doesn't file income tax returns or pay income taxes. All money that is made is considered your income. The record keeping is simple. You don't need a federal identification number for your business if you work as a sole proprietor. You may use your social security number.

Sole proprietorships are so easy to set up and maintain that you may already own one without knowing it. If you are a freelance writer, a massage therapist who is not on an employer's payroll or a salesperson who receives only commissions, you are already a sole proprietor. Even though a sole proprietorship is easy to start and maintain, you may have to comply with local registration, business license or permit laws to make your business legitimate.

limited liability companies (llcs)

In order to create an LLC, most states require two owners, who can be spouses. An LLC is set up like a sole proprietorship in that all the profits go directly to the owners, but there is a distinction between the owners and the business, protecting the owners from any personal liability. The paperwork for creating an LLC is less complex than that for a corporation, but more complex than for a sole proprietorship. Go to www.llc.com for more thorough information about LLCs.

corporations

Corporations provide a business entity that is separate from the owner as an individual. It can be expensive to start a corporation, but the owner avoids liability. Minimum requirements for maintaining a corporation include conducting annual meetings, filing minutes in your corporate books and filing the required documentation with the state on an annual basis. While double taxation is sometimes mentioned as a drawback to incorporation, the S corporation (or Subchapter corporation, a popular variation of the regular C corporation) avoids this situation by allowing income or losses to be passed through on individual tax returns, similar to a partnership. The main reason for incorporating is to limit your personal liability. You would pay yourself a salary.

setting up a sole proprietorship

Unless you have a strong business background and are up for the task of creating a corporation or LLC, we recommend starting your business as a sole proprietorship. You can always transition to another kind of business structure in the future, but for your first year as a health counselor, a sole proprietorship will likely provide you with everything you need.

After you have made certain the business and domain names you want are available, you may fill out a simple DBA form with your local government. A DBA, which stands for "Doing Business As," is a business filing that allows business owners to operate a company under a name other than their own name at a minimal cost. In most states, if your business is your first name and last name, such as Jane Smith Health or Healing with Jane Smith, a DBA is not required. However, if you want your business to be called "Holistic Healing," you will need a DBA since that business name is not your legal name (Jane Smith). Having a DBA allows you to use a name without filing a legal entity, such as a corporation, partnership or LLC. It also protects the business name from being used by anyone else. Most states and counties require that you file a DBA to legally run a business by a name other than your own, even a small home-run business. Also, banks won't let you open a business account unless you have registered your business name.

Generally speaking, the process of filing a DBA is simple and takes no more than an hour. Here's what you need to do:

- Call your county clerk's office to learn about the local fees and procedures in your area. Your county clerk can tell you where to get the DBA form, also called an Assumed Business Name form, and where to submit it.

- Follow the instructions provided by the county clerk, submitting the proper form and filing fee.

- Once your DBA filing is approved, you will get your Business Certificate. Your business is officially registered! You can now start using the name as your official business name.

Some states, such as California, also require that you publish an announcement in a local newspaper with your business name. The following website has information on the rules and regulations in each state around filing a DBA: www.businessnameusa.com/dba/state/new_york.htm.

obtaining a federal identification number

If you set your business up as a corporation, partnership or LLC, you will need to obtain a federal identification number. When you research how to register your business in your state, you will probably find instructions on how to do this. But in case you don't, you can simply fill out Form SS-4, Application for Employer Identification Number, available at www.irs.gov/pub/irs-pdf/fss4.pdf, and mail or fax it to the IRS Service Center in your state. You can also apply by phone ("TeleTIN") by calling 1-800-829-3676.

You will not need a federal identification number if you are setting up your business as a sole proprietorship. As mentioned above, your social security number will serve as your ID.

The government assigns federal identification numbers in order to keep track of small businesses for tax, budget and census purposes.

Your state's website will have information on how to select a business structure as well as the specific regulations for each option in your area. Visit the website (e.g., www.newyork.gov, www.connecticut.gov, www.newjersey.gov) and search in the "Business" section.

You can also contact the U.S. Small Business Association website at www.sba.gov for more information on the advantages and disadvantages of each business entity mentioned above, and to find a Small Business Association in your area.

Other local assistance options include Small Business Development Centers, SCORE (Service Corps of Retired Executives), Veterans Business Outreach Centers and Women's Business Centers. Look in your local phone book for any of these organizations.

You may also want to consult with an accountant, lawyer or anyone else you know who is knowledge-able about your state's laws and your personal situation.

satisfying all state and local requirements

Once you have registered your business and, if necessary, gotten a federal identification number, you will need to make sure that you are complying with all state and local requirements for running a business. For example, you may need to purchase a business license from your county. Your county's website will most likely have the information you need to make sure you are complying with coun-ty requirements, and you can use your state website to find out how to satisfy state requirements.

setting up a domain name

Next, you will want to make it easy for potential clients to find you. As an Integrative Nutrition student, you will automatically receive your own beautiful website with information about your program offerings. This saves you the expense of designing a website. We will host the website we give to you for free for at least one year after you graduate. The address of your website will be something like: www.integrativenutrition.com/graduates/YOURUSERNAME.aspx.

If you want to have a different web address, or if you want to create your own website, you will have to purchase a domain name (also known as "URL") from a provider, and have it routed to your IIN-provided website.

The benefits to having your own URL are:
- You can have your business name match your website
- The website name will be easier for people to remember

If you decide to purchase your own URL, we suggest that you go to www.networksolutions.com and follow the instructions there. There are other companies that sell domain names, such as www.register.com and www.godaddy.com. Network Solutions cost more, but oftentimes our students have problems with the cheaper companies when they try to use their new domain name with their IIN-provided website.

If buying a domain name at this time feels like too much work, you do not have to do it. Your efforts are better spent working towards doing Health History Consultations. Do not waste time figuring out how to build a complex website before you have your first five clients. If you happen to be a web designer or know someone who would do this for you at minimal cost, then it may be worth it.

business bank account

We find that it is helpful to have separation between business and personal finances. Some small business owners pay business expenses out of personal accounts and deposit business income and income from other sources into family checking accounts that are shared with a spouse. While this may be okay in the beginning, as you grow your business, not having one bank account for business and one for personal or family expenses can create complications.

For example, if you do business under a name other than your own, your bank may not allow you to deposit checks that are made out to your company name. And if you have your business money in a joint account with someone else, what happens if you have to write a check for your business the same day your husband, wife or partner drew on that same money for something else the same day? Also, if you keep your business money in your personal account, when it comes time to do taxes, it will be more difficult to figure out your deductions, fees, expenses and so on.

As we explained, if you have a sole proprietorship, your money and the business's money are one and the same. It is not necessary for you to keep a separate business account, but it is helpful nonetheless. If you keep your business finances separate from your personal finances you can put all the money you make from health counseling into a different account and pay all your business expenses from the same account. Having a separate business account will ensure that you keep track of how much money you are putting into and getting out of your business. It will also help you when it comes time to do your taxes.

Once you register your business, you will get an official Business Certificate and you will be able to open a business bank account. If you set up as a sole proprietor and get a DBA, you will have your Business Certificate when you leave the county clerk's office. Most banks require that you have a Business Certificate to open a business bank account.

Many banks offer free checking for small business owners. You can also usually get a no-fee debit or credit card. Figure out how many deposits and how many payments you expect to make a week. Chances are it will only be a few per week, in which case you will be able to get a low-cost or free bank account. A basic plan usually has unlimited checking each month.

Find a reputable bank that you have used in the past. It's probably easiest to use the same bank you use for your personal account if it has a business branch. You can call them, schedule a visit or drop in to find out what your options are when it comes to small business bank accounts.

In order to open a business bank account, you will need the following documentation:
- your federal identification number (if you are a sole proprietorship, that's your own social security number)
- a photo ID (either a driver's license or a passport)
- your Business Certificate

accepting payments

Most of our students are very skilled counselors; they are great listeners who are intuitive and genuinely enjoy talking to people. Counseling is the easy part for them. The hardest part is asking their clients for money. We will be examining this more thoroughly in Chapter 5.

To help you overcome any fear about asking people to pay you, we are going to be very clear about the different options you have when it comes to getting paid. You have two main questions to ask your clients:

- will they pay in full up-front or in monthly installments?
- will they pay using cash, check or credit card?

getting paid up-front vs. in monthly installments

Of course, it is always exciting to get paid in full at the beginning of your program. When you first start out as a health counselor, you may keep your fees low as you get your feet wet. So paying in full may be quite doable for your clients. However, as you get more experience and raise your rates, your clients may want to pay in monthly installments. We'll discuss how to price your program in Chapter 5, but to get started we generally recommend charging $95 per month while you are a student, and $195 per month once you graduate. You might consider encouraging your clients to pay in full by offering them a discount for doing so. For example, "save 10% if you pay in full" or "get $100 off the full price if you pay in full."

Some graduates actually prefer to have their clients pay in monthly installments. This helps them with budgeting. Also, the monthly payments help them to stay motivated and interested in their clients. If your client pays in monthly installments, you will need to set up a system for keeping track of the payments. An example of a very simple system is below:

Client Name	Jan	Feb	Mar	Apr	May	Jun	July	Aug	Sept	Oct	Nov	Dec
Jane Smith		$95	$95	$95	$95	$95						
Joan Evans				$95	$95	$95						
Joe Doe					$95	$95						
TOTALS		$95	$95	$190	$285	$285						

As you get new clients, simply add them to the list, and then enter each payment into the appropriate cell. Using this system, you will know how much you've earned each month, and at the end of the year you can easily tally the total income you've earned.

cash, check or credit card

cash: Everyone likes to get paid in cash. However, if you are not skilled at money management, this may not be the best way for you to get paid. Cash is easy to spend because it goes into your wallet and you forget that it was your paycheck from your client. Also, if your rates go up, it may not be feasible or convenient for your clients to pay you in cash. If your client wants to pay with cash, they should pay up-front. If they say they will pay you in cash each month, you will have to remember to ask them for the money at your sessions. You don't want to be discussing money during the program. You want them to either pay you in full up-front, give you post-dated checks or give you a credit card that you will charge each month.

check: Checks are a great way to get paid. Unlike credit cards, you will not have to pay a fee for accepting a check as payment. We highly suggest that you ask your clients who want to pay you by check to give you six post-dated checks—one for each month you will be working together. That way, you will not have to ask your client for payment each month, freeing you up to focus on what's really important in your work with them. Have your client date the checks for the same date of every month. The 1st and the 15th are usually easiest for convenience. Once you receive the checks, be sure to keep them in a safe place. Keeping checks from all clients for a certain date in one convenient spot will make your bank runs easier. It is good customer service to deposit checks within three days of their date.

credit cards: While credit cards may be very convenient for your clients, you will need to pay a fee each time you accept payment that way. We highly suggest that you start out just accepting cash and checks, and then move to credit cards once you have several clients and you have enough income to offset the transaction fees of accepting credit. The easiest way to accept credit cards is to use PayPal. PayPal lets you accept credit cards, bank transfers, debit cards and more—at some of the lowest costs in the industry. Plus, your customers can pay you instantly, even if they don't have a PayPal account, via American Express, MasterCard, Visa, Discover and debit cards. You do not need to pay any set-up or cancellation fees, and you get transaction rates as low as 1.9% + $0.30 per transaction. See www.paypal.com for details.

Another way to accept credit cards is to set up a merchant account through your bank. If you already have a business account, your bank may be able to help you accept credit cards as well.

Finally, many of our graduates use www.practicepaysolutions.com to set up an online account that accepts credit cards. With Practice Pay Solutions (PPS), you simply collect the credit card information from your client, log into the PPS website and enter in the information to charge the client. The money is then transferred from the client's credit card directly into your business bank account. If you choose this route, take a look at the credit card authorization form we've included in this chapter. Also, PPS gives Integrative Nutrition students a discount. We will be talking about this more in class.

credit card authorization form

I, _____, hereby authorize _____to charge the following credit card account in the amount shown below for monthly health counseling services. This payment agreement will be in effect until services have been completed or are ended by request of the client either verbally or in writing.

CREDIT CARD INFORMATION:

Card Type: _____ Visa _____ MasterCard _____

Card Number:	_____
Expiration Date:	_____
Name on Card:	_____
Billing Street Address:	_____
City, State, Zip	_____
Email address:	_____

Amount:	$	per month for 6 months = $	Total

Cardholder's Signature: _____

Thank you.

managing finances

A critical part of managing a business successfully is having a system and structure in place for managing your finances. This is important for tax purposes, making financial decisions, collecting payments and projecting financial goals long-term. Poor financial planning will decrease your income, and will jeopardize the success of your business. Accounting is simply a process of tracking what you spend and what you make. This also allows you to be well prepared for tax filing.

Steps for financial planning:

Step 1: Set Up a System to Track Your Finances

As mentioned, opening a separate bank account facilitates ease of tracking. Next, choose a method of tracking. Here are three options:

- use a spreadsheet or database program on your PC or Mac
- keep a ledger and record manually
- purchase a software system, like Quicken or QuickBooks

Keep on top of this work. You should plan to spend time each week updating your records. It is also important that you keep all of your receipts and tax forms from year to year, since you could be asked by the IRS to show proof of your earnings and expenses.

Step 2: Track Your Expenses

A great thing about health counseling is that you won't have many large expenses. No inventory, no employees. The biggest expense you will have is rent, if you are renting an office space, and your client giveaways. We suggest that you spend approximately 10% of your client revenue on giveaways. So if your client is paying you $200 per month, you have $20 each month to spend on gifts.

Per tax regulations, you are eligible to deduct expenses for your business from your income. These expenses must be "incurred in connection with your business, ordinary (similar to others in your field), and necessary." Basically, any money you spend to run your business can be deducted, either in whole or by percentage. Your accountant will know the specifics and the regulations.

You should track all items, whether you paid cash, check or credit card. Keep every receipt, and organize them by category in a large manila or accordion envelope. If you had no receipt, record the amount, item and date with whatever system you have in place.

These are the types of expenses you may want to include:

- all goods you purchase for clients—books, CD-ROMs, tapes, food samples, self-care items
- office equipment—computer, fax, copy machine, phone, chairs, table, frames, plants, lighting
- business use of home or rental office – you are entitled to deduct the percentage you actually use for seeing clients and running your business
- business supplies: paper, CD-ROMs, pens, files
- email, Internet and computer costs

- phone bill—you may deduct a percentage, based on how much you use your phone for business
- marketing and promotion—ads, flyers, brochures, networking event fees, business cards, website creation, designer fees, hiring people
- insurance (renters and liability)
- legal and professional services
- continuing education—workshops, seminars, events related to your field, learning a complementary modality (check with accountant what is legal)
- entertainment—taking clients to dinner or to event (a percentage is deductible)
- event expenses for clients—such as the cost to rent a room for a workshop or food purchased for a cooking class
- transportation and lodging—including speaking engagements, out-of-state conferences or business meetings
- association fees, including the The American Association for Drugless Practitioners
- bank fees
- car—lease or purchase payments, gas, mileage related to business travel (you may deduct a percentage, based on how much you use your car for business)
- if you rent an apartment and your office is in your home, a percentage of your rent may be deductible

In terms of what you spend on Integrative Nutrition tuition, tax law states that education expenses incurred to change careers are not deductible. Education expenses that are extending your knowledge of your current profession are deductible, based on IRS guidelines. Again, your accountant will know what and how much you can deduct of expenses. As noted, some items are only a percentage, not the full amount. Laws vary from state to state.

Step 3: Track Your Revenue
You should record all income you earn related to your business—cash, check and credit card payments.

Types of revenue from health counseling:
- client fees from your program
- speaking engagements
- group program revenue
- corporate workshops
- income from writing
- consulting income
- referral fees given to you by other practitioners

Track this revenue in your ledger or with your software, organizing it by month and by client. By using a software program, it makes it much easier to add, analyze the figures, and to have a detailed and organized record to give to your accountant.

If you have other income from your day job, you should also keep accurate records for this, and provide all of the income to your accountant who will be able to properly prepare your tax forms.

Step 4: File Your Taxes

We recommend that you set aside 30% of your income for taxes. For example, if you collect $200 from a client, set aside $60 for taxes.

It is important to note that the tax laws are very complicated. And while this book is meant to provide an overview of financial planning, it is not meant to take the place of a qualified accountant. By spending money on an accountant, you actually save money, since he or she will know exactly how to provide the greatest savings for you and your business. Being self-employed means that you have the chance to keep a large percentage of what you make, since you are allowed to deduct expenses for your business. And tax laws are designed to support businesses.

If you really don't want to hire an accountant, you can purchase tax preparation software, such as Turbo Tax.

another word about money

Usually when people go into business for themselves, issues about money come up. After all, this may be the first time in your life when you are directly asking people to pay you for your time. It is a common belief today among certain people that in order to be spiritual you cannot make or have a lot of money. Letting go of this belief and realizing that you can have abundance in your life will help you tremendously in your health counseling. What you are offering your clients is incredibly valuable, and you deserve to get paid well for it. It's important to get very clear on your ideas about money so that you do not create blocks for yourself when it comes time to get paid.

money belief system:

What are your earliest memories of money?

_____

_____

_____

_____

_____

_____

What were/are your parents' views of money?

_____

_____

_____

_____

What do you enjoy about money?

_____

_____

_____

_____

What difficulty do you have around money?

_____

_____

_____

_____

What is your current relationship with money?

_____

_____

_____

_____

_____

_____

For further reading about issues with money, we recommend *Creating True Prosperity,*
by Shakti Gawain, New World Library $13.95.

typical money personalities

Throughout the years, we have identified that our students fall into different categories in terms of their relationships with money. Take a moment to see which one you identify with. Get support around letting go of any troubled past with money and recognizing that you can have a future full of abundance and wealth.

- **the under-earner:** These people do not want to charge or charge very little for services. They believe this should be free to everyone. They usually ask for about $25 per month for their six-month program. These students have extreme difficulty raising their rates and asking clients for money.

- **the over-giver:** These people doubt their abilities as health counselors and make up for their insecurities by over-giving. They often spend a lot of money on giveaways and food. Their sessions usually go longer than the allotted hour. They spend a lot of what they earn on their clients and end up with little profit. These people need to recognize how healing their presence and support are.

- **the over-spender:** These people wish to portray themselves as successful. They spend lots of money on upscale offices and expensive clothes to help themselves feel professional and cover insecurities about doing this work.

In all these cases, remember that your financial health and your belief in your own self-worth are tremendously important. The truth is that however you approach money in your career as a health counselor is how you approach money in all areas of your life. If you take this opportunity now to form a healthy, balanced relationship with money, it will change your life. By keeping yourself financially healthy, stress is usually reduced, which contributes to your overall health and happiness.

professional liability insurance

Be sure to have all your clients sign the legal waiver that we provide you on the CD-ROM. After you graduate, you may want to purchase professional liability insurance if you can afford to do so.

Prices for professional liability insurance may range from $250 to $500 per year. Two organizations that offer professional liability insurance are:

- The American Association for Drugless Practitioners: www.aadp.net. (After you graduate, if you become a member of AADP, you can purchase practice insurance from them.)
- Healthcare Providers Service Organization: www.hpso.com.

We have never heard of any of our graduates needing professional liability insurance, and you can legally practice without it. Whether or not you purchase it is up to you.

business plan

A business plan is an organizational, financial and clarification tool that will aid you in moving your business forward. In your business plan, you will clarify your goals and thoroughly think through how to accomplish them.

A business plan can be very simple or complex. Here is a formula for a simple business plan:

First, decide how much money you want to make from health counseling over the next year. Write that here: _____

What would that work out to, on average, per month? _____.

Next, figure out what you want to charge for your services. Most of our students start out at $150 per month while they are still in school. After they graduate, they typically increase their rates to $195 per month. From there, rates can go to $250 per month, $295 per month and higher. (We'll discuss raising your rates in Chapter 10.)

How much do you want to charge your clients each month? _____

Now, divide how much you want to make each month by how much you want to charge your clients each month. This is the number of clients that you will need to pay you each month to reach your income goal. Write that here: _____
(Example: You want to earn $24,000 from health counseling this year.
Which means you want to earn $2,000 per month.
If each client you work with is paying you $195 per month, you will need to have 11 clients to pay you each month.)

From here, you can plan how many Health History Consultations you will need to do each month.

On average, 50% of your Health History Consultations will become clients. This percentage will improve as you get more experience, but this is a good number to use starting out. So if you want to get four new clients, you will need to do eight free consultations. If you do eight free consultations each month for three months, you should have 11 clients.

The next step is to determine how you will get eight people to come in for free Health History Consultations. We'll talk in later chapters about how you can do this by giving public talks, networking and other methods.

Eventually, you may want to create a more detailed business plan. There is a great outline for creating a business plan on page 370 of *Business Mastery* by Cherie Sohnen-Moe.

check-in

We've just given you a lot of new information about how to start a business as a health counselor. And there is much more ahead. The next chapters will show you how to get out there, sign clients and be successful. Right now you may be feeling excited or nervous, overwhelmed or confident. Wherever you are is totally fine. Remember to stay focused, follow our instructions and ask for support when you need it.

Take a minute to check in with yourself. How are you feeling about your business? What have you accomplished so far? What has been the most challenging part? What are you most looking forward to?

_____

_____

_____

_____

_____

_____

_____

_____

_____

_____

_____

_____

_____

_____

Before I came to Integrative Nutrition, I was an actor turned massage therapist. I wanted to add another dimension to my massage practice, where I could use my mind and voice rather than just my physical body. Also, my massage clients were always asking me health-related questions. I wanted to give them answers and get paid for my expertise.

Adding health counseling to my massage practice was easy. I offered all of my clients free Health Histories and many of them signed up for my six-month program. I also invited friends, family and everyone I met for Health Histories. People were genuinely interested and eager to hear more about what I do.

A month before graduation I had four clients, and I set a goal to have more before the school year ended. Within weeks of setting my goal, I had three more clients. The school gave me the motivation, support and skills to make it happen.

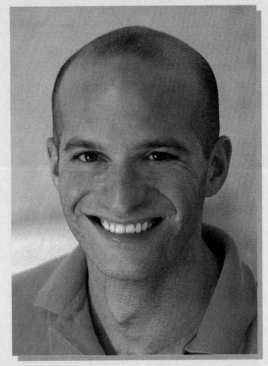

Larry Rogowsky
Bronx, NY
larryrogo@hotmail.com
2006 Graduate

The whole concept of building your business while still in school is brilliant. I really encourage you to start your business now while you have tons of support so you can be on track when you graduate. It's important to take consistent action. Set attainable goals, make a clear plan to achieve them and take small steps daily.

Because my office is located in the theater district, I work with many performers, as well as busy profes-sionals. I help them to slow down, take time to eat and take care of themselves. I teach my clients to choose foods that give them the sustainable energy their lifestyle demands. I work with them to achieve optimal health and be the best they can be at all times. My first few health counseling clients have spread the word about me, so my business is growing mainly through referrals. Health counseling re-energized my massage practice too. I enjoy massage more now that it is not the only work that I am doing.

Now that I'm cooking and eating whole foods, my own health is much better, my energy is great, and I'm inspiring my friends and my partner. Life has changed on many levels. I've met incredible people and have built really strong relationships.

I love that we are on the cutting edge of the health industry. I am making a real difference in peoples' lives by being myself and using my strengths of humor, care and love. I have the freedom to be flexible and put my personality into this work. I love sharing information and ideas and empowering my clients to decide for them-selves the choices that are right for them.

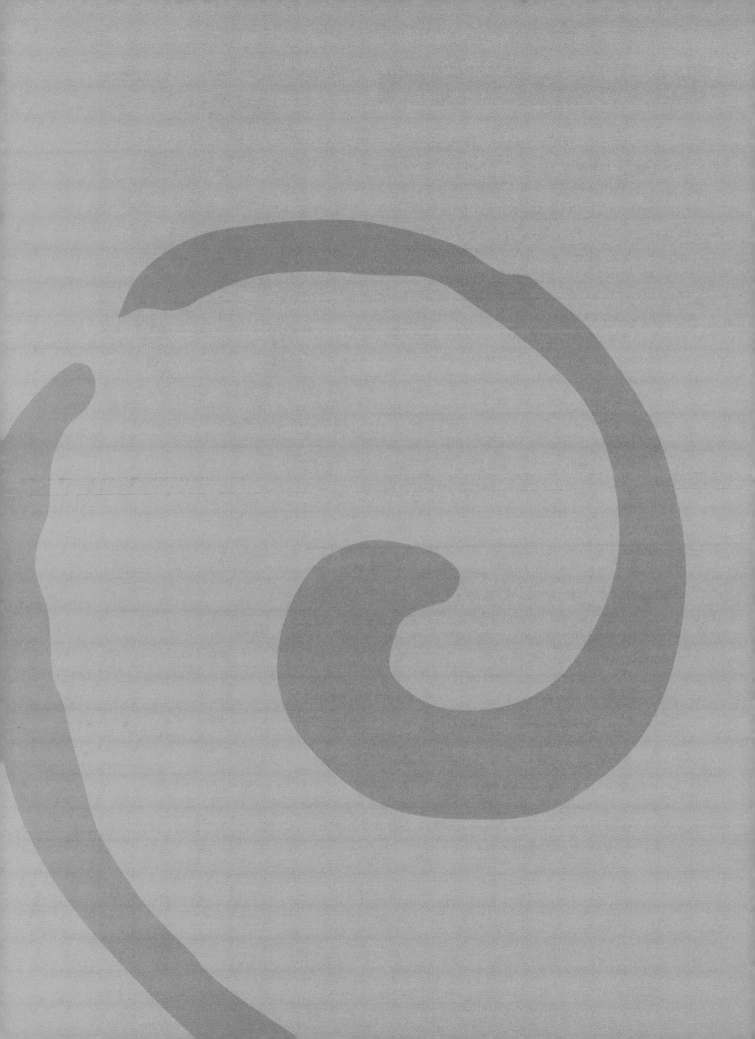

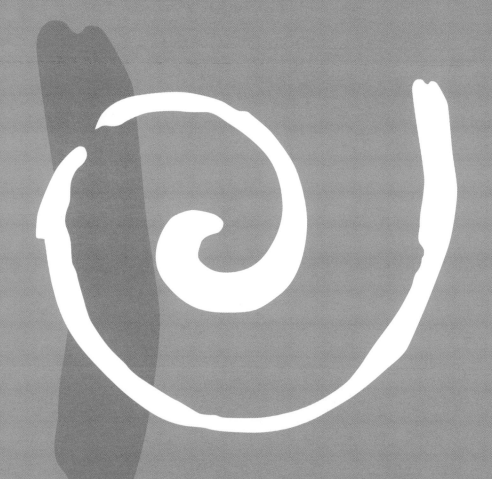

chapter four

In order to succeed, your desire for success
should be greater than your fear of failure.

Bill Cosby

getting clients

many of our graduates have such large numbers of clients come their way that they need to hire additional health counselors to help counsel all their clients. Wouldn't it be great if you were attracting so many clients you didn't know what to do with all of them? In order for you to get to this point, you have to put in a lot of work and practice doing Health Histories, workshops, marketing and networking. Even if you think you are not good at or don't like marketing yourself, this chapter—and the curriculum taught in class— will support you in finding ways of marketing yourself that best suit you. Once you figure out how to attract the clients you want, you will be able to focus on building your business.

target market

In the early stages of health counseling, we recommend you do Health Histories with almost anyone who is interested, excluding people who are obviously problematic or suffering from life-threatening illnesses. As you do Health Histories with all different types of people, you will naturally start to identify the types of people who are attracted to you and those who you most enjoy working with. For example, maybe you notice you really enjoy working with new moms. From there, you can narrow your marketing efforts to focus on getting Health Histories with new moms. You can ask yourself, where can I go to meet new moms? What are the concerns of new moms? How can I create an email or flyer that will address those concerns? New moms then become your target market. Other target markets might be busy executives, college students, marathon runners, yoga instructors or people with a specific health concern (such as celiac disease, candida, migraines, sleep problems, stress or weight loss).

benefits to having a clear target market:
- it is easier to market your services when you know who you are trying to reach
- you can become an expert in a few particular health concerns, rather than learning about new health concerns with each new client
- people want to go to health practitioners who are experts in whatever their health concern is
- you will enjoy health counseling more if you are working with people who are interesting to you
- people in this target market most likely know a lot of other people like them who will also be ideal clients for you.

Answer these questions to help you identify your target market.

1. What health or life issues are you working on or have worked through? Your own experience and expertise may make you a perfect health counselor for people who are experiencing something you've already been through.

_____

_____

_____

_____

_____

2. What type of person would you take pleasure in working with? Perhaps you've noticed in your Health Histories so far that a particular type of person really connects well with you, and you with them. You can list a few different types of people here. Get as specific as you can, e.g., women with eating disorders, single dads, twenty-something people who live in New York City, women going through menopause, people with diabetes, children ages six to 10 or corporate professionals.

_____

_____

_____

_____

_____

3. Out of these groups, who can afford your six-month program fee?

_____

_____

_____

_____

_____

4. Now that you have identified people who you would like to work with and who can afford your services, where can you find them? For example, working mothers may spend time at day care, or be involved with working mom groups or school functions. You can go to the places where your target client hangs out, and share with people what you do as a health counselor.
(See information on networking later in this chapter.)

_____

_____

_____

_____

_____

_____

5. What are the characteristics and qualities of people in your target market?

Age range _____

Male or female _____

Education level _____

Career _____

Income _____

What are their needs, concerns and goals? _____

Who else serves these people? _____

_____

Once you have identified the type of people you are trying to reach, you can narrow your networking and marketing efforts. This allows you to more effectively design and write your materials, as well as improve how you communicate what you do.

If you want more help on this subject of target markets, see page 271 of *Business Mastery*, by Cherie Sohnen-Moe.

dynamic introduction

As you probably already know, one of the basic steps to getting clients is to clearly communicate what you do. After all, how can people become clients if they don't know what you do? You should be able to summarize everything that you do in one or two sentences. This is what we like to call your "elevator speech."

Here is the formula for a powerful elevator speech:

My name is _____

I am a health counselor. I work with _____

who _____

Fill in the blanks.
The first blank is your name, obviously. The second blank is your target market. The third blank is what you help your target market with.

For example:
My name is Jane Smith. I am a health counselor. I work with young professionals who want help incorporating regular exercise, healthy foods and stress management into their lives.

OR

My name is Jane Smith. I work with busy moms who want to learn how to prepare healthy meals in under 20 minutes that their families will enjoy, while also making sure they have a high level of self-care.

OR

My name is Jane Smith. I work with men who are addicted to sugar to help them balance their blood sugar levels, incorporate health-promoting foods into their diets and reduce sugar cravings.

company mission statement

After you've identified your target market, you can develop a mission statement for your business. A mission statement is a sentence, bullet points or paragraph illustrating the goals and purpose of your business. It's the vision of your company put into words.

qualities of a powerful mission statement:
- states your purpose
- has a central theme
- is accurate and succinct
- includes a description of the services offered
- includes a description of your target market
- focuses on a few key attributes of your services

examples of mission statements

Disney: To make people happy.

FedEx: FedEx is committed to our People-Service-Profit Philosophy. We will produce outstanding financial returns by providing totally reliable, competitively superior, global, air-ground transportation of high-priority goods and documents that require rapid, time-certain delivery.

Saturn: Our mission is to earn the loyalty of Saturn owners and grow our family by developing and marketing U.S.-manufactured vehicles that are world leaders in quality, cost, and customer enthusiasm through the integration of people, technology, and business systems.

Integrative Nutrition: We want to help evolve the future of nutrition by encouraging, cultivating and promoting healthy foods and a balanced lifestyle. At our school we teach fundamental and practical knowledge of traditional and modern approaches to nutrition, East and West. Our students learn how to effectively share this important, life-changing information with friends, family and the general public. Our students become empowered to reach out and touch many lives. Integrative Nutrition is committed to the idea that if we all stand up and speak up for what we know to be true, a ripple effect will occur that will dramatically improve the healthcare system in America, and throughout the world.

As you can see, mission statements range from very simple to more complex. Some companies include their target market and/or their ethical position.

some examples of health counseling mission statements might be:

Jane Smith Health provides busy moms with support in maintaining a healthy family and a high level of self-care.

As a health counselor, my mission is to improve the health and happiness of all my clients.

Use this space to write a first draft of your company mission statement. This is just a first draft; it need not be perfect. You can always refine it as your business grows.

_____

_____

_____

_____

_____

Use this mission to guide you. Your mission will be a powerful motivational tool for you, keeping you clear about the bigger picture of why you are doing what you are doing and what is driving you to accomplish your goals. Whenever you are unsure what steps to take with your business, think back to this mission statement and ask yourself, will taking this action support the mission of my company? Also use your mission to help you reach your target market. By speaking clearly and confidently about why you are doing the work you are doing, people will become interested in you and want to learn more.

dress to impress

The importance of maintaining a professional image cannot be emphasized enough. How you present yourself to the world sends a message about how you view yourself. One way to send out a message that you are professional is to dress that way. This does not mean that you need to wear a business suit every day. It means that you ought to dress in a way that makes you feel good about yourself and reflects your work as a health counselor. If your target market is yoga teachers, wearing a business suit to a workshop is inappropriate. Likewise, if your target market is corporate professionals, wearing flip-flops and jeans is not the first impression you want to give. You want to dress in a way so that people in your target will be drawn to you, relate to you and also see you as competent. You also want to be comfortable and confident in your clothing.

Keep in mind that you never really know where your next client might be. You could meet him in the grocery store, at Starbuck's, at a restaurant or on the train. For this reason, consider dressing to impress every time you leave the house.

marketing materials

When you go out and meet potential clients you'll want to have marketing materials that convey who you are and what you do. We will provide you with business cards, brochures and a website to get you started. While you are a student, we want you to focus on doing Health Histories, not spending your precious time and money at your computer designing marketing materials.

As your business grows, you may eventually create your own logo, color scheme and style for your marketing materials. The look and feel of these materials should be consistent with how you want people to experience your services. For example, if you work primarily with women, you might want your marketing materials to feature lighter colors and more feminine images. If you work with male athletes, you'll want your materials to have a stronger, more masculine quality.

To get a high-quality logo, you can hire a graphic designer. A good graphic designer will work with you to understand what you want the image of your business to represent. Through this process, the designer will show you some options for logos. He or she may also help you pick out colors and fonts for your business and design your business card. Before hiring a designer and agreeing to the fee, you should get very clear on what exactly you are paying for. How many drafts of your logo do you want? Usually, this kind of work demands three drafts: the first draft illustrates brainstorming about look, feel and colors; the second draft shows the direction you have chosen; and the final draft is tweaked to get it exactly as you like it. It can cost $300 to $1,500 for the design of a logo. If you know a skilled graphic designer you could barter with, that may be a good option.

Alternatively, you can use an online service, such as Vistaprint, that has a selection of logos. You can pick one that works for you and create your own business cards, brochures, notepads, postcards and more. Using such a service, you can also upload your own original logo onto these materials and print them out.

here are examples of some marketing materials:

• Business Cards: Your business card will represent you long after you have given it away. The front of your card should include your name, title (e.g., Health Counselor), company name, telephone number, email address, website address and logo. You can also include your physical office address and fax number. The back of the card can be used as well. Here you can have a cool design, an inspirational quote, a tagline or a listing of your services.

• Brochures: A brochure is a great "leave-behind"—something you can take with you to networking meetings or give out at talks. Your brochure should match your business card in look and feel, and can include parts of your core mission: who you work with, the concerns they have, the benefits they get from working with you and what makes your services unique. You should include your name, title, company name, address, phone number, email address and website address. You may also want to include a short section that describes who you are, including your educational background and training. You will receive a predesigned brochure from Integrative Nutrition. In addition, a company such as Vistaprint can help you create your brochure, or you can create your own using software such as Microsoft Word or PowerPoint.

• Your Bio: Your bio is a few sentences of background information on who you are and what you do. You may have a couple of versions of your bio that you can use in different circumstances. Your bio should include pieces of your mission, such as who you work with and how you help them. It should also include your educational background and any special trainings or certifications you have.

• Press Kit: A press kit is a collection of marketing materials that you can give to people you meet. You can also send it to companies, yoga studios or centers where you would like to do workshops. Your press kit can be very simple. A two-pocket folder, with a slot on the inside for your business card, can hold all the contents of your press kit. Inside you can include:

- your bio
- your brochure
- a workshop flyer
- your business card
- a description of your services
- a list of workshops that you do
- anything else you think is important
- an outline of one of the workshops that you do
- an introduction letter to the person you are contacting
- an interesting and relevant article that you or someone else wrote

• Website: When you are ready to create your own website, it will expand on your core mission even more than your brochure does. It should match your other marketing materials in terms of look and feel. Pages to have on your website might be: Home, Who We Work With, How We Help, Services, About Us, Success Stories and Free Stuff. The Free Stuff page can offer any articles you've written, recipes or back issues of your newsletter. The Free Stuff page is a great marketing tool—a way to get people to linger on your site a little longer than they might have otherwise. There are many online website host companies that provide templates for new websites. As mentioned in Chapter 3, we recommend Network Solutions (www.networksolutions.com) as we have found that our students have minimal issues with them.

successful networking

Building your business is about building relationships. The more people you meet and know, the more likely you are to find prospective clients, or to create the possibility of having clients referred to you. Understanding and practicing networking will help you grow your business and spread the word about who you are and what you do. The larger your network of friends, colleagues, contacts and acquaintances becomes, the better your chance of success. People like doing business with people they know. As you become increasingly recognizable as a health counselor, you create what we call VFT.

- Visibility—being seen
- Familiarity—the more often you are in contact with people, the more they remember you and your services
- Trust—being reliable, responsive and knowledgeable fosters this

Networking is a way to expand the circle of people who you know and who know you in order to increase the buzz about your business. Think about it. If 100 people know that you are a health counselor and then they each tell one person who tells one person about you, your chances of getting a phone call are dramatically higher than if only 20 people know you are a health counselor. And if 1,000 people know you are a health counselor, your phone will ring even more!

Simply put, networking is talking about what you do to as many people as possible. There are many benefits to networking, such as:

- becoming known in your community as an expert in health and nutrition
- getting new ideas from others on how to provide your services and how to build your business
- creating the opportunity to schedule more Health Histories
- building referral systems with other professionals
- adding people to your contact list for all of your communications, emails, newsletters and workshop announcements
- having fun by meeting other people and learning about who they are and what they do

where to network

You can network anywhere: on the train, at the gym, at a restaurant or in a more formal networking atmosphere where everyone is there for the same reason. Here are some places you might want to think about networking.

- Networking groups – There are specific groups that exist for the sole purpose of bringing people together to make contacts and help one another build their businesses. Some of these groups include Business Network International (BNI) (www.bni.com) and National Women Business Owners (www.nwboc.org).

- Associations or organizations in your field – There are a lot of different groups organized for people who are interested in health and nutrition. To find out where some of these might be in your neighborhood, you'll have to do a little research. You can ask around at gyms, yoga studios and schools, and read the paper to see if there are any groups already in place. These are a great place to share with other counselors and nutritionists, especially those with different target markets. Also, if you have another area of interest or hobby, attending meetings with those people and talking about your new work as a health counselor is a great idea because you will already have something in common with them.

- Trade and professional groups that your target market attend – Many professions have associations and groups to which they belong. For example, if you are interested in working with women business professionals, you could attend various networking events for those women in your area.

- Trade and professional groups that your referral partners are likely to attend – Referral partners are critical to growing your business, whether they be doctors, chiropractors, yoga teachers, hair stylists or personal trainers. They each belong to and attend events based on their professions. You can attend these events too, get to know them, and let them get to know you!

- Lectures, workshops and conferences – There are conferences on every topic, from health and healing, sports and entertainment to arts and crafts, exercise and finances. Find out when these events happen and attend them. You may even want to lead a workshop. There is more information about workshops later in this chapter.

- Social, cultural or sporting events, including mixers and parties – You never know when you are going to meet a potential client or referral partner. When you start health counseling, it is helpful for you to be social, to see people who you haven't seen in awhile. You could get clients at your high school reunion, by meeting up with an old friend or meeting new people when you are out.

- Charity events and fundraisers – You may want to donate a Health History, a cooking class or even a three-month program to a charity to help increase your visibility. When you attend the event, you can tell people that you donated your services, and that will start a conversation about what you do as a health counselor.

• Chamber of Commerce – Your local Chamber of Commerce hosts various events and workshops. Contact them, and find out their schedule.

Where do you think you could most successfully network your services?

_____

_____

_____

_____

_____

_____

_____

_____

_____

_____

Once you have identified the types of events you think will be most beneficial to attend for building your network, you'll want to contact the organizations that host them. Here are some ways to find specific organizations if you don't already know where they are located.

• Chamber of Commerce—They have multiple listings of events in your area. Visit or call for information.
• Yellow pages.
• Newspapers and magazines—Various events, social outings and group gatherings are advertised in the paper.
• Online—Most major groups publish their information online. Go to Google or Yahoo, type in a search and see what comes up!
• Specialized publications that your target market reads—There are publications on every topic imaginable, from pets to medicine to teen health. Find these publications, read the event listings and contact key people.
• Ask other people who are knowledgeable—Talk with successful friends, colleagues and co-workers about where they network and what they suggest. Get to know people who are successful in business and find out how they network.

create a networking calendar

What groups, associations or organizations have you researched? When are their events?

Group _____

Event Date _____

Event Time _____

Location _____

When You Will Go _____

Group _____

Event Date _____

Event Time _____

Location _____

When You Will Go _____

Group _____

Event Date _____

Event Time _____

Location _____

When You Will Go _____

Group _____

Event Date _____

Event Time _____

Location _____

When You Will Go _____

how to network

The following steps will help you become a successful networker:

- Do the research and find out what is happening in your area, with your target market and with your referral partners. Use the steps above and make a list of all the events and groups you can find.
- Contact the groups, associations and people you've researched. Get a copy of their calendar and ask questions about their events and members.
- Pick a couple of networking groups related to your niche market, hobbies and interests. Use the networking calendar you created above and start to attend events. Try them on.
- Networking is like dating; you may not click with every group you attend, but you are gaining valuable experience in the process. Try different groups and see which one feels right.
- Start your own group. A great way to network is to contact people you know who also have their own business and are looking to make contacts. You can meet once a month or so, and have tea or breakfast or lunch. Get to know each other better and share ideas on business building. Begin to refer to others in your group and ask them to refer clients to you. Great people to include are doctors, lawyers, business people, acupuncturists, massage therapists, hair stylists and accountants.

networking tips for introverted people

- Take a small step outside your comfort zone. Even researching events is a great beginning.
- Be patient.
- Get support.
- Invite an extroverted friend with you to the event. They can introduce you to people and help you feel more at ease.
- Introduce yourself on the phone to the event leader, and go to tea with them as a first step before diving into the group.
- Volunteer. This is a perfect opportunity to help others and meet people.
- Use our tips for good conversation skills and ice-breakers for small talk.
- Speak to the people you feel most drawn to.
- Avoid large groups that are intimidating, instead speak to 1, 2 or 3 people at a time.
- Start by asking others questions about what they do. Get them talking, and they will enjoy being listened to. Then, either they will ask what you do, or you can tell them.

networking mistakes

- talking too much
- lack of eye contact
- asking for business, being pushy
- showing up in casual, sloppy clothes
- only hanging out with people you already know
- forgetting to offer or invite people to do anything
- going to the event hungry and eating the whole time
- focusing on getting clients rather than building relationships

when attending a networking event

- Start talking to people, especially those you are drawn to, or ask the event organizer to introduce you to a few people. The more people you meet and add to your contact list the more likely your business will grow. Be passionate about what you do; people know when you are sincere. Use your elevator speech.
- Use a firm handshake, look people in the eye, make a good connection. Pin your nametag on your right side so it's more visible when you shake hands.
- Listen, be friendly, show interest in others; use the verbal skills you've learned at IIN on starting conversations and communicating effectively.
- At events, select a few "key" people to align yourself with. Organizers and promoters usually know most of the people, and they can be a great resource for you. You could even volunteer at an event and introduce yourself to all the attendants.
- Always give people your business card. Give the promoters your card too.
- Get everyone else's cards. Have an organized way to keep track of the business cards you collect as discussed in Chapter 1, using a business card folder, Rolodex or online tracking system. Make notes on the back of the business cards about the people you meet so you remember what you talked about and how to follow up with them.
- Be gracious. Ask people you meet to put you on their mailing list. Show them you are interested in what they do.
- When you get home that night or the next day, record the contact information of the people you met. Keep track of them—remember, it's VFT. Subscribe them to your newsletter (only if you've asked for their permission and they've given it). Send them a follow-up email. You have to be proactive and take the initiative to contact others since they probably won't contact you.
- Try to attend at least two networking events per month. Be patient and persistent.

Networking and building a business take time, and it's okay to make mistakes. Just remember to keep moving forward!

workshops

Leading workshops is one of the best ways to get clients. It is also a great opportunity for you to practice being in front of the room and to strengthen your communication skills. By teaching a group of people topics related to health and nutrition, you will really start to become an expert. Your confidence will increase and you will begin to acknowledge how much more you know about health than the average person.

In the beginning, aim for getting five to 10 people in a workshop. As you build your public-speaking skills and expand your business, you can lead workshops for increasingly more people. The idea is to attract the types of people who you want as clients. You can present at community centers, libraries, health food stores, women's groups, schools, universities, health centers, wellness centers, gyms and even your own home.

When you approach a new location about doing a workshop, it is always helpful to visit the location in person, introduce yourself and ask who is in charge of programs or scheduling. Once you are talking to this person, indicate that you are looking to volunteer to do workshops to help the organization. Tell them your elevator speech and ask, "How can I help support you by bringing in more people to this location and offering my expertise to the community you serve?" Play the role of a health counselor. Make the workshop a win/win situation for both you and the location.

We suggest that you bring your press kit with you when visiting potential workshop spaces. You can include an outline of your proposed workshop in the press kit, along with a page full of positive feedback you've collected from participants at past workshops (if you have this).

workshop marketing

You don't have a workshop unless you have participants. So marketing your workshop is essential. The following are ways to promote your workshop.

- Post flyers at key locations, like health food stores, community centers, bookstores or any locations where your potential target market spends time.
- Tell everyone you know about the workshop—clients, friends, family and colleagues. Have them tell people and offer them a referral incentive.
- Send an email announcement to your contact list.
- Mention the workshop in your newsletter.
- Invite people from the organization where you are giving the workshop. Encourage them to invite people internally and in their announcement board or newsletter.
- Go to other events and make yourself known. Hand out flyers at expositions, social gatherings, health fairs and similar events.
- Post on websites—yours or websites of any of your referral partners.
- Take out an ad in a publication that your target market reads.
- Place an announcement in the events listing section of local newspapers or newsletters.

It's a good idea to ask people to sign up for your workshop in advance so that you know who is coming. You can do this by having them RSVP to you or to the location that is holding your workshop. If you have people RSVP to the location, be sure to give the location a sign-up sheet that they can use to keep track of your participants, including names, telephone numbers and email addresses.

presenting the workshop

The workshop begins long before the actual start time. Familiarize yourself with the outline and handouts we gave you on the CD-ROM for the Sugar Blues talk. If you are creating your own workshop topic, use that outline and format to design your own workshop. Or you can use the template provided below to create an agenda. Practice your talk on your own at home or for friends. Find an assistant, someone to come with you as your support person.

The day before your workshop, send a reminder email out to participants. Then make sure you have everything you need, including:

- workshop outline—you may want to print this out in a large font size so that it is easy for you to read
- your assistant to provide support, pass out handouts and help schedule participants for Health History Consultations
- your business cards
- a sign-in sheet
- a sign-up sheet for Health History Consultations with actual time/day slots that you are available—prepare this before the workshop by referencing your calendar to find times when you can do the sessions
- handouts related to your talk
- snacks/food to give out (fruit, trail mix, simple treats)
- a watch in case there is not a working clock at the location

The day of the workshop:
- set up
- exercise
- eat well
- center yourself
- go over your outline
- arrive at the location 30 minutes early

conducting the workshop
- Greet guests warmly.
- Have everyone fill out the sign-in sheet. Your support person can help with this.
- Start strong and share information about yourself so attendees can relate to you. Share why you do this work or something about your own journey. Tell a story. You may want to share how you came to be interested in nutrition. All this helps you be real to your audience.
- Follow your outline. It's okay to go on a short tangent or to incorporate ideas not on the outline, but use the outline to guide you and keep you focused.
- Use humor when appropriate; it helps people feel comfortable.
- Bring props, something to catch the participants' attention. It could be an ad for unhealthy food from a magazine or a box of sugar. Pick something that feels right to you.

- Don't give all of your information away. Talk more about what's "wrong" than about tips on what to do. If you say too much, attendees will not be as inclined to want to work with you. For example, talk about the health consequences of eating too much sugar, not necessarily how to stop eating sugar.
- Be interactive. Use paired shares and group shares, and call on people.
- Have giveaways and handouts that participants can take with them.
- Connect participants to the concept of how difficult it is to be unhealthy. Call on one volunteer; ask them to share the pain of being unhealthy and how it has affected their life and health. By doing so, you make that person and all participants more aware of their current situation, and they in turn may realize that they need guidance to feel better.
- Share examples of client successes at appropriate times.
- Stop for breaks—stretching, questions.
- Share goals. Ask participants what they would like to make happen in their lives. Have them share this verbally or write.

ending the workshop

- Do a paired share and have participants talk about what they learned at the workshop, one thing they will take with them.
- Leave enough time to talk about your program, explaining what you do while sharing the value of working with a health counselor.
- Use a call-to-action technique. Remind participants that real change comes from taking action; so now it's time to take action towards the goals they mentioned in the workshop. That comes by first signing up for a free Health History. Also, tell them if they go home and think about it or don't sign up in the moment, it's more likely they will just stay stuck. You are offering a free hour of your time to discuss their goals more deeply, and explore how you would support them in your six-month program to create a truly amazing life.
- Have your assistant sign people up for Health History Consultations, using the sign-up sheet you created. Write the date and time of each consultation on the back of your business card, and hand these to Health History clients.
- Give your card to all workshop participants. Thank them for their active participation.

follow up

- Send thank-you emails to participants; appreciate them for their time.
- Add everyone's contact information to your mailing list.
- Send a confirmation email to Health History clients to remind them of their session time.
- Send some type of email handout related to the content of your workshop to each participant. When you give something extra after the workshop, participants see you as a valuable and knowledgeable support person.

top 10 ways to get clients from your lectures

1. Bring food. Nothing attracts participants to your workshop like free food. This is a way for them to taste the types of foods they could expect to learn how to make, and also gives them something tangible to grasp.

2. Tell client success stories. Try to sprinkle your talk with several stories of success. For example, "When one of my clients, a busy mother of three, came to me, she was totally hooked on sugar. These days, after adding some of the tools I described, she is much more energized without the need for sweets." Clarify what the problem was before and how you helped that person. This presents you as a problem solver and gives you credibility. If you have no clients to talk about, think about the health concerns you've overcome or the people you've helped over the years.

3. Make your talk interactive. Don't talk at them, talk to them. Encourage interactive elements such as paired shares, group shares and group exercises. People love to talk. They are much more likely to be interested in your talk if you include them.

4. Do a mini-counseling session demo in front of the class. Not only does this establish your credibility and expertise, it gives the participants an idea of how you work and your style of counseling. If they like what they see and the results you have with your counseling demo, they will be inspired to sign up with you.

5. Collect useful contact information. Be sure to have participants sign in and share their email and mailing address. This is a great opportunity to invite them to receive your email newsletter. Even if they don't sign up for a consultation, you can add them to your newsletter and they will remain on your radar. When they think of nutrition and wellness, they will think of you.

6. Provide a valuable giveaway. You want them to go home with a useful tip that they can refer to often, with your contact name on it. You can give away a favorite recipe that's related to your talk, tip sheet, special report or article. Perhaps they will pass it on to someone who is interested, or simply think of you when they use it.

7. Bring an assistant. Bring a classmate, a buddy or someone who loves and supports you. Let your assistant handle the logistics of signing people in, collecting contact info and scheduling Health Histories for you. If you need anything, they can support you. This will give you time to mingle and interact with participants, and it also makes you look very professional. Alternatively, you can bring a client who's willing to share the benefits of working with you as a testimonial.

8. Make sure the audience knows what you do. Many times people do not sign up for a con-sultation because they have never been asked. Leave time in your talk to introduce your services. Remind yourself that what you offer is an opportunity. Otherwise, it's just another lecture full of tips that they will never use. The best way you can help them is to offer them your program. You also want to leave time at the end of your talk to mingle and answer questions.

9. Circulate an evaluation form. Sometimes people are shy or just need to think about things. A great way to get feedback on your talk is to create an evaluation form. Ask what they liked, learned and enjoyed. Ask what future topics they would like to hear. Most importantly, ask if they would like to learn more about one-on-one health counseling and when would be a good time to call. Be sure to include space for a phone number and email address. We provide you with a sample evaluation form on the CD-ROM.

10. Make sure attendees have a way of contacting you after the lecture. Put a brochure, business card and/or your bio on each person's chair. It gives them something to read when they arrive and helps them be clear on who is giving the talk. Get used to giving your materials out like hotcakes.

overcoming nervousness

You might be nervous about giving a workshop. That's totally normal. In fact, public speaking is often the biggest fear our students face. It's one of those times where you'll have to feel the fear and do it anyway. By the end of the year, most of our students become comfortable and confident public speakers, and it is one of their favorite aspects of this work. Here are some helpful tips on overcoming the fear of public speaking.

Prepare: The more you prepare, the more comfortable you will be with your workshop. Plan ahead what you want to talk about by making an outline. Consider what objectives you want to have for your workshop. What do you want your audience to get out of it? For example, you may want them to leave your workshop with an ability to identify hidden sugars in foods. You almost always will want them to sign up for a Health History Consultation with you. Once you know your objectives, you can create an agenda to meet those objectives. Your agenda becomes a roadmap. When you create your agenda, think about how much time you will allot to each topic you will cover, as well as how you will conduct that part of the workshop (e.g., a lecture versus a paired share or group activity) and any materials or handouts you will need. Here is an outline template that you can use to create a workshop agenda:

workshop objective:

What You Will Cover	How	Timing	Materials Needed

Breathe: One of the best things you can do to stay grounded and focused when leading a workshop is to breathe. Use the paired shares and group shares as a time for you to check in with yourself and make sure you are breathing and relaxed.

Start small: If you are very nervous about leading a workshop, you may want to start small. You can invite three or four friends over for a workshop in your home. You can practice with them and ask them for feedback, what you did well and what you could improve.

Realize that everyone wants you to be successful: Anyone who comes to your workshop is there because they want to learn from you and have a positive experience. They are on your side in that they want the workshop to go well just as much as you do! Understanding this and believing it will go a long way towards helping you relax into your role as the workshop facilitator.

newsletter

Your newsletter is a fundamental part of your health counseling business. It is a relatively simple way for you to get information out to a lot of people at one time. It can be part of the Free Stuff section of your website, or a free giveaway that you offer during networking and as part of your six-month program. Also, writing your newsletter is an educational and creative outlet for you. To write a good newsletter, you'll have to pick a topic interesting to you and do a little research. Then you get to let your personality come out and write it in a way that expresses who you are.

To help you with this, we have provided you with several newsletters on the CD-ROM to get you started. You can use these newsletters just as they are, tweak them to make them more "yours" or write your own, using them as idea generators.

there are several ways to send out your newsletter:

Snail Mail – This is an option. However, we do not recommend it because of the high costs involved (printing, mailing) and the trouble of addressing the envelopes.

Email – You can simply copy your newsletter into the body of an email and create an email distribution list. This option is okay at first if you only have a few people to send your newsletter to, but you will quickly grow out of this.

Yahoo Group – Some health counselors choose to send their newsletters out via a Yahoo chat group. The advantage of this method is that people can sign up for your newsletter via Yahoo, and you do not need to personally manage the distribution list as you would if you were just sending out an email.

Online Newsletter Service – There are several online newsletter services that you can use to send out your newsletter. Webvalence (www.webvalence.com) and Constant Contact (www.constantcontact.com) are two examples. Webvalence costs about $25 per month. They have templates that are easy to use, or you can design your own. You simply copy or type your newsletter into their website and schedule it to be sent at a certain time. Constant Contact is more expensive and offers more in terms of tracking your recipients. Once it goes out, you can track who read your newsletter, when they read it and what links they clicked on (if any). If you have a website, you can add an email newsletter sign-up box to it so that visitors can easily register to receive your newsletter.

health fairs

Many health counselors use health fairs as a way to increase their visibility in the community. It can be a public health fair or a private fair for a business or an organization. You can find out about health fairs by talking to other health practitioners or by signing up with a health fair organizer. Most of these organizers are local, so ask around to find one in your area.

At the fair, you will most likely have a table or booth to display your business. Here are some things you might want to bring with you to the fair:

- brochures
- business cards
- sign-up sheet for your newsletter
- tablecloth (unless one is provided for you)
- large sign with your business name on it
- sign-up sheet for free Health History Consultations
- some kind of free giveaway—food samples, tea, organic chocolate
- bouquet of pretty flowers in a vase to draw attention to your table
- some kind of drawing opportunity—people fill out a small questionnaire with their name and contact information and get entered into a drawing for a free month of health counseling, a book, a basket of healthy goodies, etc.

I work full time leading a global logistics team in export transportation. A year ago, I was operating on autopilot, going into the office early and staying late every day. I would visit doughnut shops and the vending machines daily, and grab dinner at any place that was still open at 10:00 pm. My weekends were spent recovering, preparing for another week of the same. A major health problem created a turning point in my life and an opportunity to take an honest look at myself. Integrative Nutrition appeared at exactly the right time.

During the school year, I took control of my health and stress level, while creating a part-time business that sings to my soul. With the skills and confidence I gained at Integrative Nutrition, I was able to establish healthy boundaries at my job. I was able to get out of my own way, take control of my schedule and prioritize my work more effectively so I am not burning myself out.

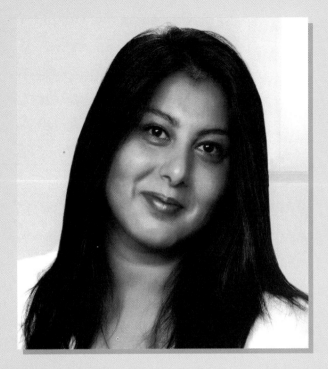

Maya Bhagat
Bloomfield, NJ
WellBeingPrana@aol.com
2006 Graduate

I got my practice started by doing Health Histories and Sugar Blues talks over and over again. My first talk was at a holistic health center, with an audience of five or six people. They didn't seem to pick up on my fears, and one person signed up immediately for the program. From there, I booked talks at Whole Foods, the YMCA and the Girl Scouts. I kept doing talks, breaking through my fears around public speaking and becoming more comfortable each time. News of my business spread through these speaking engagements, and I continued getting Health Histories and new clients. By the time I graduated, I had 11 paying clients.

Through my experience doing talks, I've learned that it's just as easy and much more effective to book a series of talks rather than one at a time. This way I am doing less marketing and saving time. I do monthly talks at the YMCA on various health topics, and I recently completed a three-part lecture series for the Girl Scouts, with more planned for the future.

A beautiful thing I learned at the school is that when someone doesn't sign up for my program or book a talk, it doesn't mean I'm a bad person or that I'm not good enough. I ask myself what I can try differently next time instead of staying paralyzed in rejection or defeat. It's much more empowering to see these situations as opportunities to learn and grow.

I was amazed by how much business information the school provided. They present a banquet of choices, where you can pick and choose what tips and techniques to use. The tips are simple, specific and strategic. The school has really figured out how you can get the most results from your effort, so trust in the process and take action.

I have come so far in such a short period of time. It's astounding what you can accomplish during the school year, so jump in and use all the resources and support to make an amazing career and life for yourself.

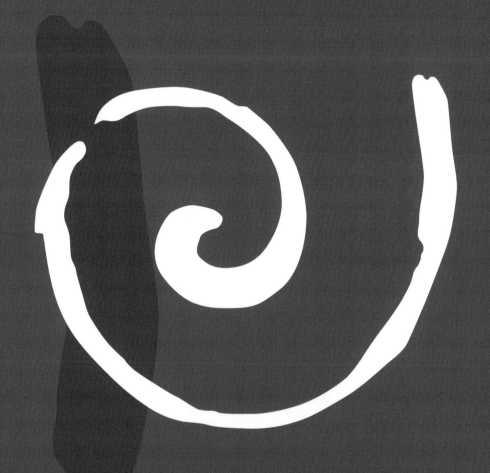

chapter five

If you hear a voice within you say
"you cannot paint," then by all means paint,
and that voice will be silenced.

Vincent Van Gogh

closing the deal

typically, people attracted to health counseling are intelligent, unique, intuitive and generous. It is very common for them to have difficulty asking for money. If you want to be successful as a health counselor, you will have to overcome blocks around money and your value. We will support you with this throughout the year, but the best way for you to learn is to simply practice closing the deal. Closing the deal—the part at the end of the Health History where you ask your potential clients if they want to work with you—comes easily to some people, but for most people it is the most difficult part of the Health History. In this chapter, we will walk you through the different aspects of closing the deal and provide you with information and tools on how to do this successfully.

ending the health history

After you go through the Health History form, leave about 10 to 15 minutes to close the deal. As we mentioned in Chapter 2, here are some steps to take:

- Mention one thing you enjoyed about your potential client and the session.
- Ask them, "How was this for you?"
- Ask them, "What was one thing you found valuable in our session?"
- Restate some of the person's health concerns and the three things they know they could be doing for their health that they are not doing.
- Explain in detail what they get from your six-month program (At this point, you may want to get out your Program Agreement, which clearly lists everything that is included in your program. Sometimes having a visual of all this information is helpful.):
  - two one-hour appointments each month for six months, which will include discussion of the client's progress, recommendations and a full set of notes
  - monthly special events like a health food store tour and group discussions related to health and wellness
  - an invitation to bring guests to the special events
  - a variety of handouts, recipes, books, CDs, foods and other materials
  - email support in between sessions
- Let them know that all of this is included in your monthly fee.

- Ask them, "Does this sound like something you might be interested in?"
- Ask, "Do you have any questions?"

    They will probably ask how you accept payments.

    Explain that they can either pay in full or in monthly installments.

    Explain that they can pay via cash, check or credit card (if you take credit cards).

example of specific language for explaining program cost

"The program is $150 per month, and that includes everything: our meetings, monthly seminars/cooking classes, books, CDs, my newsletter, a health food store tour and email support in between sessions. But if you register today, you'll save $25 per month."

bonus

For those of you who are really comfortable with asking the questions above, you can ask a bonus question: "Do you know anyone who might be interested in doing a Health History with me?" If they say yes, get that person's name and find out the best way to contact them.

power statements

The following statements are useful tools for you to close the deal successfully, wrapping up Health Histories in a way that will make potential clients more likely to sign up. Use these as you like and feel free to adapt them to your style.

- During the six months that we'll be working together, I am committed to teaching you a set of skills you will be able to use for the rest of your life.
- When we begin to work together, I think a perfect place to start would be (three things identified in the Health History).
- We would work together for the next six months, which gives us time to get to know each other and to make slow but lasting changes.
- I could give you a list of 25 things to do and you would probably do them for a week—and then the list would go under the bed with the dust bunnies.
- We would check in with what is going on with you and see how the recommendations went from our last session.
- You would always leave with a list of recommendations to put into action in the two weeks between our sessions.
- Much of the program is driven by you, and no two programs are the same. Each one is completely individualized, based on your goals, your needs and the pace at which you want to go.
- In addition to our 12 sessions, I support you with books, materials, recipes, food samples and handouts that enhance the changes you are making.
- When do you think we could start working together?

the program agreement

This Program Agreement is a document that you will give people once they say they want to sign up for your program. It contains your program offerings, price, disclaimer and a legal waiver. There is a copy of it on your CD-ROM.

program agreement

It is a pleasure to welcome you to this Program. During the upcoming six months, you will learn ways to help yourself achieve a healthier lifestyle. Please read the following. If anything is unclear, please ask.

This Agreement is made today between the Counselor of the Program, and the person named at the end of this document, [the Client]. The Program in which you are about to enroll will include all of the following:

A. Two one-hour appointments each month for six months, which will include discussion of your progress, recommendations, and a full set of notes

B. Monthly special events like a health food store tour and group discussions related to health and wellness

C. An invitation to bring guests to the special events

D. A variety of handouts, recipes, books, CDs, foods and other materials

SCHEDULING

I understand that my clients have busy schedules and I take pride in not keeping them waiting or keeping them longer than planned. Each session will end an hour after it was scheduled to begin. Please be on time. If the Client needs to cancel or reschedule an appointment, please do so **24 hours in advance.** Otherwise, the Client will forfeit that appointment and not have an opportunity to reschedule it.

Program begins _____ And ends_____ ("End Date")

This program expires if all 12 sessions have not been completed within two months after the End Date specified above.

PAYMENTS & REFUNDS

The Client understands that the regular cost of the Program is $195 per month for 6 months. However, registration today reduces that cost to $150 per month. Upon commencement of the Program, the full amount of $900 is due and must be paid in full. However, in order to assist the Client to afford this Program, the Client may pay for Program Fee in monthly installments by credit card or a series of post-dated checks. If the Client selects to pay in full, then the cost shall be reduced by another $100 total (for a total cost of $800).

In the event of the Client's absence or withdrawal, for any reason whatsoever, the Client will remain fully responsible for the unpaid balance of the Program. Under no circumstance will the Counselor refund any payments made by the Client. By signing this Agreement, the Client agrees to be legally obligated to pay the full amount of this Program.

DISCLAIMER OF HEALTHCARE-RELATED SERVICES

The Counselor encourages the Client to continue to visit and to be treated by his/her healthcare professionals, including, without limitation, a physician. The Client understands that the Counselor is not acting in the capacity of a doctor, licensed dietician-nutritionist, massage therapist, psychologist or other licensed or registered professional. Accordingly, the client understands that the Counselor is not providing healthcare, medical or nutrition therapy services and will not diagnose, treat or cure in any manner whatsoever, any disease, condition or other physical or mental ailment of the human body.

The Client has chosen to work with the Counselor and understands that the information received should not be seen as medical or nursing advice and is certainly not meant to take the place of your seeing licensed health professionals.

PERSONAL RESPONSIBILITY AND RELEASE OF HEALTHCARE-RELATED CLAIMS

The Client acknowledges that the Client takes full responsibility for the Client's life and well-being, as well as the lives and well-being of the Client's family and children (where applicable), and all decisions made during and after this Program.

The Client expressly assumes the risks of the Program, whether or not such risks were created or exacerbated by the Counselor. The Client releases the Counselor, his/her heirs, executors, administrators and assigns, his/her officers, directors, shareholders, employees, teachers, lecturers, agents, health counselors and staff (collectively, the Releasees) from any and all liability, damages, causes of action, allegations, suits, sums of money, claims and demands whatsoever, in law, admiralty or equity, which against the Releasees, the Client ever had, now has, or will have in the future against the Releasees, arising from the Client's past or future participation in, or otherwise with respect to, the Program, unless arising from the gross negligence of the Releasees.

CHOICE OF LAW, ARBITRATION AND LIMITED REMEDIES

This agreement shall be construed according to the laws of the State of [your state]. In the event that any provision of this Agreement is deemed unenforceable, the remaining portions of the Agreement shall be severed and remain in full force. In the event a dispute arises between the parties, either arising from this Agreement or otherwise pertaining to the relationship between the parties, the parties will submit to binding arbitration before the American Arbitration Association (Commercial Arbitration and Mediation Center for the Americas Mediation and Arbitration Rules). Any judgment on the award rendered by the arbitrator(s) may be entered in any court having jurisdiction thereof. Such arbitration shall be conducted by a single arbitrator. The sole remedy that can be awarded to the Client, in the event that an award is granted in arbitration, is refund of the Program Fee. Without limiting the generality of the foregoing, no award of consequential or other damages, unless specifically set forth herein, may be granted to the Client.

If the terms of this Agreement are acceptable, please sign the acceptance below. By doing so, the Client acknowledges that: (1) he/she has received a copy of this letter of agreement; (2) he/she has had an opportunity to discuss the contents with the Counselor and, if desired, to have it reviewed by an attorney; and (3) the client understands, accepts and agrees to abide by the terms hereof.

Counselor name _____ Signature _____ Date_____

Client name _____ Signature _____ Date_____

As soon as people agree to sign up for your program, hand them this form and give them a moment to read it over. We recommend that you state out loud your cancellation and refund policies, as well as the disclaimer that you are not a doctor. You want to be certain that your client understands these important details.

You must have all your clients sign this Program Agreement. Without it, there is no contract between you and your client, meaning your client could back out of the program at any time. Being clear about the Program Agreement is in your best interest and the best interest of the client. Some clients will want a copy for their records, so bring two copies to each Health History.

scheduling clients

As soon as your client signs up for your six-month program and you both sign the Program Agreement, pick the days and times that you will have your sessions. Scheduling all your future sessions at the end of the Health History will reduce the amount of back and forth you have with the client throughout their program. Use the Program Schedule on your CD-ROM to help you with this.

Fill out this form with your clients after they sign the program agreement, and give them a copy or tell them you will give them a copy at their first session. Be sure to reiterate what it says on the bottom of the Program Schedule, which is that the sessions last one hour from the scheduled start time. If clients show up late, their sessions still end on time. Also stress the importance of your 24-hour cancellation policy.

pricing your program

When pricing your program, start out with a cost that feels comfortable to you, but also compensates you fairly for your time and expertise. Inevitably, pricing your program is going to bring up issues you have around money. Please use your counselor and the OEF to get support. Our students all come from different backgrounds. Some of them are young and just out of school, and the idea of making $30 per hour is very exciting. Other students come from professional backgrounds, where they are used to making over $100,000 a year. It's important for you to acknowledge where you are on this spectrum and be gentle with yourself along the way.

We recommend students start at $150 per month, or $900 for the six-month program. Some of you may already be used to charging this much. Maybe you are a massage therapist, nutritionist, physician or private yoga instructor. If this is the case, you can charge $175 or more for your first few clients. If charging $150 a month is scary for you, then you have two options. Feel the fear and do it anyway or lower this fee. Perhaps you want to charge your first client $50 per month. If you do this, we encourage you to charge your second client $100 per month and your third $150 per month.

In general, we recommend you charge $150 while you are still a student and raise your rates to $195 to $250 after graduation. Many graduates then raise their rates to $300 or $350 after another six months or a year of health counseling. Some go on to charge $450 or even $500 per month. There are people out there who can afford these prices. It's up to you if you ask for them or not.

When setting your fees, consider how many clients you actually want to work with and how much money you want to make from health counseling this year. See the "Business Plan" exercise at the end of Chapter 3 to help you with this.

program schedule

Client name: _____

Appointment day: _____

Appointment time: _____

	Individual sessions	Group events
Month 1 _____	_____	_____
Month 2 _____	_____	_____
Month 3 _____	_____	_____
Month 4 _____	_____	_____
Month 5 _____	_____	_____
Month 6 _____	_____	_____

Additional notes: _____

_____

_____

I understand that you have a busy schedule and I pride myself on not keeping you waiting and not keeping you longer than planned. Your session will end an hour after it was scheduled to begin.

Please arrive on time. If you have a need to cancel or reschedule your session, please do so at least 24 hours in advance. Otherwise, you forfeit that session.

lower-income clients

If you want to offer your services to people who do not make a lot of money—such as young people, senior citizens or single parents—you have a few options.

You can offer a sliding scale. When potential clients ask how much your program costs, you can say something like, "I have a sliding scale from $100 to $150 per month. What works for you?" Whether these are your actual parameters or you create others, you should still feel you are getting paid fairly for your services.

Another possibility is to offer group programs. You can then charge less per person while still making the same amount of money for your time. We will discuss group programs more thoroughly in Chapter 6.

Applying for grants may work for you, especially if you want to work in schools or within certain communities.

Another thing you can do is to find a client who can afford more than your usual fee, and then put the difference towards a client who can't afford your usual fee. For example, if you charge $150 a month, but you know you have a Health History with someone who makes a lot of money, you can charge that person $250 and then offer your program to someone else for $50 per month.

discounts

People love to save money. So if you want to charge $100 per month for your program, an effective sales strategy may be to tell potential clients that your program costs $150 per month, but if they sign up today (the day of the Health History), you will give them a discount of $50 per month. You may also extend to them a reason why you are giving this discount. Perhaps it is because they are a young person or a single parent, or because you really want to work with them.

asking for money

If this chapter about money has your heart beating with anxiety, know that you will make it through. You can still become a successful business owner, even if right now you are nervous about asking for money. Here are some strategies to help you overcome your concerns and confidently ask for the money you deserve.

1. Start your practice by taking on one or two barter clients so that you become confident in the value and effectiveness of your services. Then when you start asking for money, you will be very clear about what your clients are paying for. See more on bartering below.

2. Work on clearing up your money issues in your personal life. If you have difficulty asking for money in a business setting, this issue is probably coming up in all areas of your life. Look and see, are there a lot of people who owe you money? Do you owe money to people? Do you have difficulty asking for what you want? Are you afraid of money? Do you feel that you don't deserve money? Practice asking people for money they owe you. Nurture and value the money you have. Get in the habit of happily receiving compliments, favors, gifts and money from others.

3. When closing the deal, focus on the other person, not on yourself. Learn that receiving money from your client benefits them by making it much more likely that they will reach their health goals. When you ask a potential client for money, the conversation is not about how much they value you, but about how much they value themselves. Asking your client for money is asking them to make a commitment to their own health. Paying you is an important action, symbolizing their investment in themselves and their decision to get well.

When you ask for money, all kinds of feelings may come up. Relax, stay focused and keep listening to the person. Your role is to show them everything they will get for their money and point out all the great benefits, and then support them to invest in themselves. You can point out that it is unfortunate that people spend so much money on their clothes, their cars, their houses and going out to eat, but not on their bodies, which is where they live our whole lives. You can support them to turn that around in their own lives.

4. Learn that being paid for your work helps you have a positive relationship with your client. Money is energy. In order for you and your client to build a healthy working relationship, the energy flow between you should be equal. You will be giving this person a great deal of your time and energy, not only in sessions but also when you photocopy handouts, buy gifts, teach a cooking class, etc. You can see money as the way that they send energy back to you, creating an even give-and-take so you both feel energized.

5. Know that an exchange of money for your services also helps keep clear boundaries between you and your clients. As a health counselor you will be warm, friendly and loving, but you are also a paid professional. It's important to keep this boundary clear, especially when it comes to the occasional client who misuses your time, bounces checks or treats you like their mommy, daddy or best friend. Having clear written agreements and the appropriate exchange of money helps you set limits, keeping the counseling experience positive and happy for you.

asking for money tips
- Feel your fear, and do it anyway. Don't give into your fear about asking for money, because it will make your business stagnant.
- Practice your closing the deal statement with your buddy, friends and family. Asking for money is simply a muscle that needs flexing.
- Write down all the things that could happen when you ask for money: the person could say no, the person could give you the money but resent you, if it's a friend, it could hurt the friendship, etc. Write down all of your fears to get them out of your hair.
- Always be honest. Don't answer questions that you don't know the answer to and don't promise anything that you can't deliver.
- Make sure potential clients know what they are getting for their money. Go over the Program Agreement and/or show them your rate sheet so they are clear.
- Tell a success story to illustrate what is possible if they work with you.

owning your value

Here is a story for you. One of our students, whose name was Christina, was charging $25 per month for her six-month program and wanted to charge more, but was uncomfortable doing so. She consulted a counselor, another student, to help her raise her rates. The counselor asked Christina how it was going working with her clients. Christina said it was great. She loved working with her clients and they were seeing many results. However, Christina was a dancer and really enjoyed working with other dancers. She didn't think it was fair to charge a lot for her program because she said dancers don't have a lot of money.

The counselor asked Christina about her favorite client and the benefits her favorite client received from the program so far. Christina began to list them. The client had lost 10 pounds; she moved out of her parents' house and got her own apartment; she began cooking for the first time ever; she quit a job she hated and got a new, better paying job; she entered a new, loving relationship; and she cleared up her digestive concerns. The client was also beginning to develop a spiritual practice and getting closer with her friends. And this was only the beginning of Month 4!

successful bartering

The most important thing when bartering is to make sure it is an equal trade, and that you are receiving something you want. Perhaps you'd like to trade with a massage therapist, a private yoga instructor or a web designer. A good rule to start with is an hour of your time for an hour of theirs. It's also smart to pick someone to barter with who may turn into a referral source for you. For example, pick a yoga instructor who has a large clientele. She may share some of the things she learns from you with her clients, who may then want to come see you. Other people to barter with may include hair stylists, personal trainers, chefs, life coaches, Reiki practitioners, music teachers, language teachers or writing coaches.

Even though bartering may seem casual, it is crucial that you sign an agreement with your barter clients. This will make you look more professional, and prevent your bartering clients from rescheduling, canceling or not fulfilling their part of the agreement.

*See page 190 of *Business Mastery* for more information on bartering and different bartering organizations.

positive feedback

One way to help you realize your value as a health counselor is to consistently ask for feedback. You have probably noticed that at Integrative Nutrition we ask students what they like about the calls, classes and orientations. You should incorporate this technique into your business.

At the end of each Health History, counseling session or cooking class, ask the client or participants what they enjoyed. Really listen to what they say and allow it to sink in. Also, at the end of each six-month program, ask your clients to fill out the completion form and the last session wrap-up form. Both of these documents are on your CD-ROM. Having your clients write down all the benefits they received from their work with you will help you comprehend exactly how valuable you are.

"So," the counselor repeated to Christina, "your client has cleared up health concerns, lost weight, is cooking, moved into a new apartment, got a new job and has fulfilling relationships." "Yes," Christina replied. The counselor asked, "Christina, how much would you pay someone to help you with all of that?" Christina replied, "$5,000." The counselor asked, "So, why are you charging your clients only $150 for your program?"

In reality, Christina was not keeping her prices low because dancers couldn't afford more than $25 a month. She was keeping her prices low because see couldn't see how much her services were worth.

We share this story with you because you probably have something similar going on. We know that what you have to offer is priceless. Your clients will change dramatically as you introduce them to healthier foods, primary foods and new cooking techniques. The high-quality listening you offer will change their lives.

It is interesting to note that many graduates who are charging $100 a month have difficulty signing clients. However, once they raise their rates to $200 or $250 a month, people sign up without batting an eye. This is because the counselors did not recognize their own value, so neither did the potential clients who came to see them.

If you own what you are worth, others will follow.

What Are You Worth?

1. List Everything That Your Clients Get As Part of Your Six-Month Program:

_____

_____

_____

_____

2. What benefits have your clients and/or friends and family received as a result of knowing and working with you?

_____

_____

_____

_____

_____

_____

_____

3. What makes you an excellent health counselor?

_____

_____

_____

_____

the magic of mirroring

Inevitably, when you are a health counselor, the people who come to you for your services are going to be going through a lot of similar life circumstances that you are. This is the magic of mirroring. If you are trying to lose 10 pounds, chances are most of your clients will be as well. This phenomenon is especially true when it comes to money. If you are struggling with money, you will attract people who are also struggling with money. This is one of the beautiful aspects of being a health counselor. It is through counseling others that we heal our own wounds and move forward with our lives.

If you find yourself attracting lots of clients who cannot afford your program, the best thing for you to do is examine your own relationship with money. How can you open up to receiving?

One tool that we find especially effective in helping people clear up any issues around money is the Clean Sweep document, created by Coach U. This "quiz" is a great guide to building a solid financial foundation. Go to http://betterme.org/cleansweep.html.

dealing with rejection

Like we've said before, on average about half the people who come to you for a Health History will sign up for your program. Some graduates have a higher closing rate and some have a lower closing rate. Regardless of where you fall on this spectrum, recognize that in this business you will always have to deal with rejection. It's a good idea to put a plan in place to help you cope with any feelings that come up and to learn and grow from your experiences.

Do not be hard on yourself when someone does not sign up. Maybe that person would have been a difficult client who would have caused you a lot of strife. Maybe that person was too stuck or distracted to make a commitment to change at this time. Maybe it's not so clear as this, and you are left wondering if you could have done more.

Whatever the situation, when someone doesn't sign up after a Health History, ask yourself what you might have done differently. Were you focused on the person and listening as deeply as possible? Could you have used more power statements? Do you need more verbal kung fu practice? Do you need more confidence when asking for money? Write down what you learned and what you want to do better next time. Then take a deep breath and move on.

It is very normal to have emotions come up when someone turns you down. You might feel sad, angry, guilty or frustrated. Remember that you are probably feeling this way because of things that happened to you a long time ago. It has very little to do with the wonderful, caring, intelligent person you are today. The only thing that has happened is that someone has chosen not to work with you at this time. Acknowledge and then let go of your feelings. Journal, make some art, go for a run, whatever works best for you. As time goes on you will come to understand that a certain level of rejection is normal, and you will not be bothered by it.

After being a business owner for many years, I found myself working for someone else as a human resources manager. Although I liked the job, I was getting burnt out and dreamed of becoming self-employed again. Integrative Nutrition offered me an opportunity to create a business out of what really excited me in life.

My passion is around spirituality and personal growth. I incorporate this into my counseling practice by educating my clients about living fearlessly and becoming deliberate creators of their own lives. In addition to teaching about healthy food choices, I focus on primary food and work with clients to help them become aware of limiting thought patterns that contribute to their health concerns. I teach about the law of attraction and abundant living. Life really turns around when we change the way we think along with improving our food and lifestyle choices.

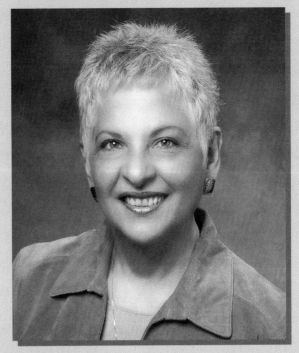

Lucia Luna
New York, NY
lucia@lucialuna.com
2002 Graduate

The first thing I did to start building my business was set up a neat and professional home office with the equipment I needed, mainly a computer and printer. Before I had any clients, I created a set schedule for health counseling in my planner. I made welcome packets, which contained the Health History Form and a brief outline of how my program works. I did all the prep work and back end office tasks as a way to create space for the clients I wanted to attract.

I made an extensive list of everyone I knew and wrote a warm letter to introduce my practice. I sent out five to seven letters in the mail per week, so I could follow up and invite them to join me for a Health History. I shared my enthusiasm for what I was up to and described to them the types of clients I was looking for. One of the first people I talked to was my family doctor because I knew she came into contact with my niche market, menopausal women. I also met with a chiropractor and acupuncturist. I offered some free sessions to the practitioners so they could understand my work and get a taste of what I did. I ended up getting referrals from the doctor, which really jump-started my business.

One of the best tips I have for closing the deal with potential clients is to make it clear that you don't work with people who aren't committed and willing to change their lives. I explain that I am running a business, and although I would love to work with everyone, I can't because my reputation depends on results. I ask them to take a minute to decide if they are ready to commit to making these changes at this point. If they say yes, I make the decision to work with them. By doing this, I consistently end up with clients who are a joy to work with and who make incredible changes.

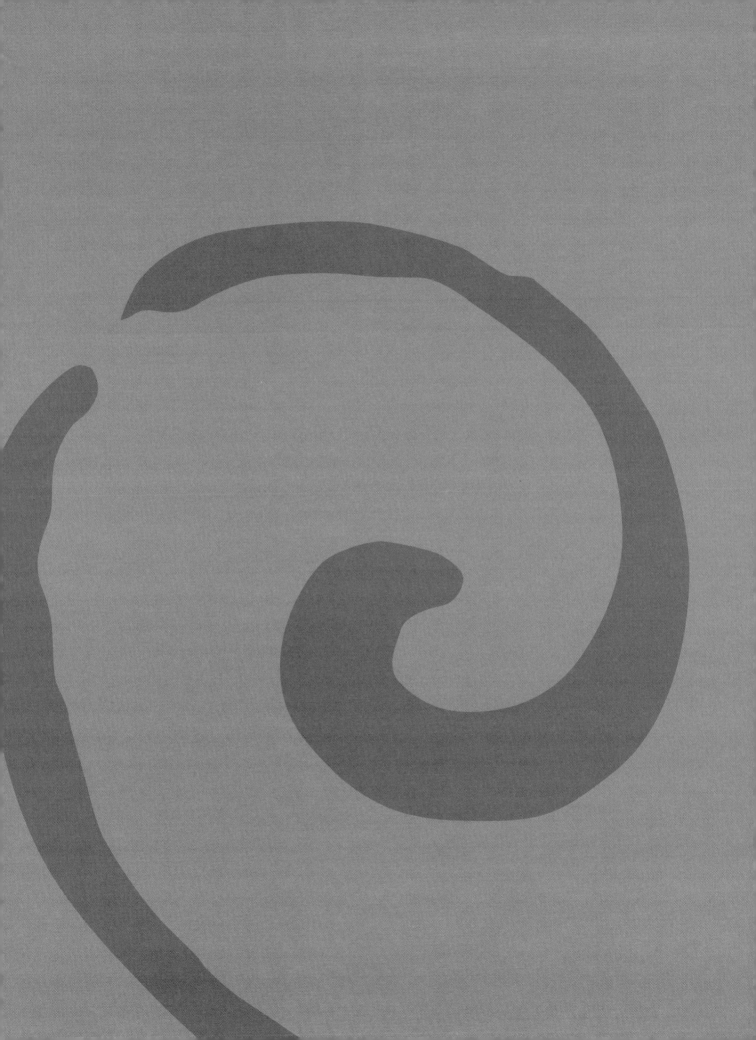

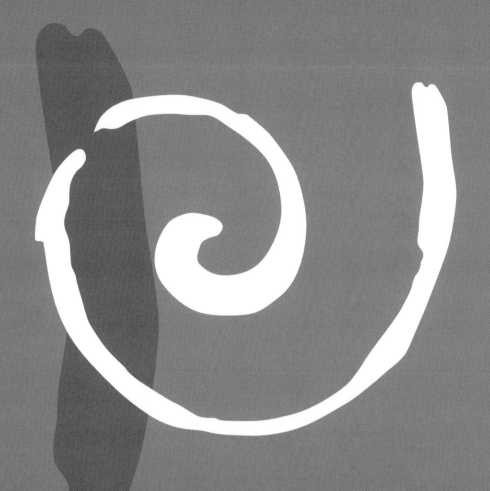

chapter six

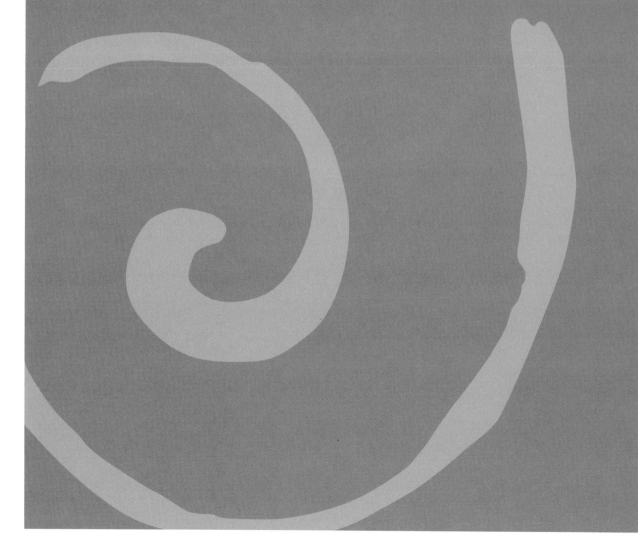

Setting an example is not the main means
of influencing others; it is the only means.

Albert Einstein

program offerings

throughout our 13 years of experience running the school and teaching people how to be health counselors, we have found that the basic six-month program meets the needs of most clients perfectly. In this chapter, we will outline the components of the basic six-month program and then discuss other options, including phone clients, teleclasses, group programs and corporate clients.

basic program

As you know by now, the following are the components of the basic six-month program:

- two one-hour appointments each month for six months, which will include discussion of the client's progress, recommendations and a full set of notes
- monthly special events like a health food store tour and group discussions related to health and wellness
- an invitation to bring guests to the special events
- a variety of handouts, recipes, books, CDs, foods and other materials
- email support in between sessions

Studies show that six months is the amount of time needed to create long-term habits. Supporting your clients for six months around making better food, exercise and lifestyle choices increases the probability that they will continue with these activities after your program is complete. The monthly events—cooking classes and monthly seminars—that are part of your six-month program are a great way for your clients to meet one another and create community, as well as an opportunity for you to meet their guests and practice your public speaking.

giveaways

One of your program offerings is the gifts that you give each client at the end of every session. These gifts need not be fancy or expensive. They may include anything from cooking utensils to tongue scrapers, from books to food. There is a giveaway checklist on the CD-ROM. We recommend you staple a copy of this to each client folder to keep track of what you have given to each client. Having a bag or a bin in your office space where you always have extra client giveaways is a great idea. That way, each time you have a client, you can look in your treasure chest and pick something out. So, when you come across a good giveaway, buy a bunch and throw them into your stash.

Here are some great giveaway items that clients usually love:

- beans
- grains
- recipes
- strainer
- thermos
- chopsticks
- water bottle
- tongue scraper
- wooden spoons
- organic toothpaste
- organic tea and a tea ball
- Louise Hay affirmation cards
- fresh greens (bok choy, kale, collards, etc.)
- *Integrative Nutrition: The Future of Nutrition*
- *The Self-Healing Cookbook* by Kristina Turner
- blank journals for writing or using as a food journal
- dry-erase markers (to write loving notes on the mirror)
- condiments (umeboshi, hot pepper sesame oil, gomasio, etc.)
- *The Integrative Nutrition Journal: Your Guide to a Happy, Healthy Life*

Most clients appreciate getting a binder in which to keep all the handouts that you give to them. You can purchase binders at Staples or other office supply stores for less than $1.00 each. You may want to tape your business card to the front or insert it inside. You can give this to your clients when they initially sign up or at the beginning of their first session. It's also helpful to give them dividers for their binder so they can create sections in whatever way that makes sense to them. Or you can do it for them: one section for session notes, one for recipes and one for handouts. This giveaway helps your clients stay organized around their self-care.

cooking classes

Teaching your clients that cooking healthy meals is easy and fun is priceless training. Most people today think that cooking takes hours of hard work. You know this is not true. Your clients will greatly value and truly enjoy learning how to cook with you.

Depending on your level of comfort in the kitchen, you may decide to offer monthly cooking classes or you may mix your cooking classes with other types of seminars. Please note that even if you do not have a lot of experience cooking, you can still teach an extremely successful cooking class. It's okay to show your clients that you are not a cooking expert, but that you still manage to make healthy meals in a short period of time. Just be yourself. Your clients will appreciate you for it.

Sample menus for cooking classes are provided on your CD-ROM.

cooking class outline

pre-preparation

- determine the date and time
- choose location
- consider travel logistics
- review cooking class menu
- watch the healthy cooking video
- find a support person (best to have a classmate)
- print out or photocopy recipes for the group
- photocopy any helpful hints or cookbook recommendations
- send reminder emails to participants (several days beforehand)

preparation – day of

- be well rested
- purchase ingredients
- prepare pots, pans, tools, etc.
- prepare ambiance (music, lights, etc.)
- bring appointment book and sign-up sheet

6:00 pm set up

- arrive early
- greet each person
- get guests' names, addresses and emails
- offer small personal introduction for those who are not already clients

6:30 pm welcome

- welcome group members
- introductions/something you're looking forward to tonight (two minutes each)

6:35 pm paired share

- something going well these days (two minutes each)

6:40 pm group share

- review menu, ingredients, techniques
- share any special cooking tips
- discuss order of preparation and cooking

6:45 pm cooking

- be sure everyone is involved in cooking
- help distribute preparation and cooking tasks
- play some fun music
- connect, cook, have fun!

7:55 pm the meal

- enjoy the meal
- share about any cooking challenges, tips and techniques
- one thing each person found interesting, fun or helpful
- make sure to especially include the quiet ones

8:20 pm clean-up

- ask for help—many hands make light work
- leave the kitchen spotless
- share leftovers

end of evening

- schedule Health Histories with those who are interested, but not already clients
- celebrate

Tips to boost your confidence around cooking classes:
- practice
- watch our cooking DVD
- attend another counselor's cooking class to watch and learn
- pair up with another health counselor and do your classes together
- make the recipe on your own beforehand so you are familiar with the ingredients and the process

Easy things to cook that your clients will love:
- quinoa
- miso soup
- soba noodles
- burdock root
- sautéed greens
- spaghetti squash
- brown rice pasta
- tempeh sandwiches
- organic turkey sausage
- roasted root vegetables
- salmon with lemon and fresh herbs

health food store tour

Many people are intimidated by the various products that appear on the shelves of the health food store. They simply buy organic or healthier versions of food sold in the regular grocery store. Some of your clients may never even have stepped foot in a health food store.

Scout out the best health food store in your area. Introduce yourself to the manager of the store. Give them your business card, explain that you are a health counselor and that part of your program involves giving your clients a tour of a health food store. Let the manager know how many people you'd like to bring on the tour and that your tour will be an hour to 90 minutes long. Explain that you'll be encouraging your clients to buy products after the tour and to come back to the store in the future to do their shopping. Most stores will be very welcoming. Ask if the manager might agree to offer your clients discounts on the day of the tour. Agree on a date and time with the manager and thank them.

Watch our Health Food Store Tour DVD and familiarize yourself with the concepts and products featured. Also, peruse this outline for ideas.

It is best not to do health food store tours between 5:30 and 8:00 pm, which are prime shopping hours. Aisles can get very congested, making it difficult for all your clients to get close to you and to hear what you are saying. The best times for health food store tours are during weekdays and after 8:00 pm.

Some of your clients may want a private tour. If this is the case, you can always substitute a health food store tour for one of their sessions. You can send long distance clients a copy of our Health Food Store Tour DVD.

health food store tour outline

early prep	find a store location to give the class ask if the students can get a discount if they buy on that day create flyers rehearse the script
preparation that day	try to be well rested, exercise and have a shower just before class bring a clipboard to use for the event sign-in sheet bring business cards, a calendar to set up appointments, and a watch to know the time
8:00 pm greeting	arrive early, check the place out welcome each person get the name, address and email of any guests
8:30 pm paired share	people continue to arrive, but start with sharing at this time "What do you want to learn today?" make sure they're all set up with a partner tell them that you'll tell them when to switch allow four minutes per person
8:35 pm group share	choose one or two people to share with the group what they shared with their partner (choose people who look alive, who have good eye contact with you)
8:38 pm introduction	start yang and strong "My intention is for this evening is to permanently change your relationship to food shopping, and for that to happen you need to be here 100% with that same intention." "Your life will turn out completely differently when you are eating well and you understand that what we eat changes everything." explain why you picked this particular health food store explain the discount on today's purchases, if you have arranged that
8:40 pm background	give a little background on your experience with health food stores the first time you were in one how weird it was and uncomfortable and how interesting

8:42
the tour
	if questions come up, answer them
	here are some points about each particular section:
	produce
	    explain how to distinguish between organic and non-organic
	    veggies
	    observe roots, greens, mushrooms, colors, shapes
	    seasonal stuff, textures, flavors, fruits
	    encourage trying new things and even
	    picking out something to take home
	    that they've never tried
	fridge foods
	    free range meats, "fake meat" (seitan, soy hot dogs, veggie turkey),
	    eggs, miso, raw nut butters, raw sauerkraut, yogurt, ghee,
	    kefir, other unfamiliar items

bulk

    grains, beans, nuts, pasta, cereal, snacks, herbs

    suggest buying these items for the first time in clear packaging so the food can be seen
    (texture, shapes, freshness), then saving packaging so they can use it again next time and
    buy bulk

packaged food

    cereal, sandwiches, grains, etc.

flours

    point out how wheat is heavy and glutinous,

    it can be hard to digest and absorb

    it isn't "bad," but there are other options

    (millet, brown rice, oat, quinoa, spelt flours)

seaweeds

    the beauty of the minerals, b-vitamins, iodine

    all are helpful, suggest experimenting with preparing seaweed

cookies + sweeteners

    how do different sweeteners make us feel?

    rice syrup, cane juice, honey, molasses

    just because it is in health food store, doesn't mean it is healthy

cleaning products

    touch lightly on supporting these companies

    (recycled, biodegradable, environmentally conscious, non-toxic)

ethnic foods

    trying new spices, sauces

    take a chance with exciting condiments

oils

    olive, safflower, sesame, canola, ghee

    suggest experimenting with different flavors, tastes, textures

    flax (not for cooking, but great for your body/brain)

tea

    relax with chamomile, digest with peppermint, warm with ginger,

    build energy with green

nutritional bars

    some are tasty, some good for extra energy,

    some are very sugar-filled like a candy bar

milks

    rice, almond, soy, enriched, goat, cow

    use them to bake, for cereal, drink hot or cold

    varieties of cheese and ice cream

makeup, health and beauty

    use clean, ethical companies

    ingredients absorb into your skin like food

    try whole food beauty products with ingredients you can recognize

herbs, supplements, homeopathy

    shifting into plant medicine

    most western drugs use plants as a base and then genetically manipulate it

    but you can try new forms of healing

    most health food stores have an expert to help you

9:25 paired share	suggest they discuss with one another something they learned and a product they would like to try
9:30 wrap up	ask people what was the best thing they got out of the tour

monthly seminars

If the idea of teaching cooking classes is nerve-racking for you, there is no need to stress. Instead, you can offer monthly seminars on other topics related to health. You can do a Sugar Blues talk or an Eating for Energy talk for your current clients. Or you can customize seminars to fit the needs of your target market. For example, if you work with corporate clients, you may want to do a stress reduction seminar. If most of your clients are busy moms, you can do a seminar on fun snacks for kids. The options are endless. These seminars are your opportunity to explore topics that are interesting to you, while simultaneously providing your clients with additional education and inspiration.

Here are some additional monthly seminar ideas:

- abundance
    - identifying limiting beliefs about money-making
    - collages about what participants want to create in their lives
    - setting new intentions about money
- creating a healthy home environment
    - clearing clutter
    - organizational tips
    - clearing negative energy (incense/smudging/salt/music)
- fasting/cleansing
    - healthy ways to cleanse
    - different forms of cleansing and fasts
    - what time of year to cleanse (springtime)
- natural beauty
    - make-your-own face scrubs
    - eating for healthy nails, skin and hair
    - anti-aging information
- slowing down for good digestion
    - benefits of stress-free mealtimes
    - creating a positive eating environment
    - chewing practice or chewing meditation
- staying healthy through the holidays
    - managing family stress
    - gift exemption
    - importance of exercise
- time management
    - identifying goals, desires and priorities
    - working smarter not harder (to-do lists/scheduling tips/delegating)
    - setting boundaries for time management
- understanding Ayurveda (or TCM, blood type diet, etc.)
    - quizzes to identify type
    - food and lifestyle recommendations
    - choose three things from this school to incorporate into diet or lifestyle

You can also offer seminars that address common health concerns. Your clients are probably hearing about these and could use some education andsupport. Health seminar topics could include:

- IBS
- allergies
- diabetes
- heart disease
- cold and flu season
- men's health issues
- women's health issues

A great way to add benefit to your program, while reducing your own workload, is to have guest speakers at your seminars. Do you know someone with their own business who could offer expert advice and demonstrate their services for your clients? They would probably be happy to speak in front of a new audience, and your clients will be thrilled to hear them. Guests will often speak for free in exchange for being allowed to give their marketing materials to your clients. Possible guest speakers include:

- chiropractors
- acupuncturists
- personal trainers
- tarot card readers
- whole foods chefs
- massage therapists
- skin care consultants
- meditation instructors
- personal finance experts
- yoga or pilates instructors
- vitamin and supplement experts

For any seminar you give, it's a good idea to create an outline first. Figure out what you want to say. Then use the talk outline for Sugar Blues or Eating for Energy to help you organize your information. Leave at least 20 minutes at the end for your clients to ask questions and get support to make specific changes based on what they just learned. Practice helping your clients to support one another. You can have them do paired shares or assign buddies to check each other's progress.

scheduling your monthly seminars

Due to clients' busy schedules, not to mention your own, scheduling can become the most complex component of your monthly seminars. At first, when you have only two or three clients, you may try to work around their schedules, but as your client base grows this will likely become impossible. We recommend that you pick one day of the week that works best for you, and tell your clients when they sign up for your program that your monthly seminars are always on that day (e.g., the first Monday of the month, the third Thursday of the month).

teleclasses

If many of your clients are phone clients, you may want to offer your monthly seminars as teleclasses. You can schedule one hour-long teleclass each month. Topics can range from cooking tips to Sugar Blues to Eating for Energy. Almost anything that can be taught in person can also be taught on the phone. your call and make it available for people to listen to afterwards.

Even if your clients are local and you hold in-person seminars, teleclasses are a low-cost, convenient way to expand your business and spread the word about your company.

There are many free or low-cost teleclass companies you can use to set up a teleclass. You may schedule your teleclass on www.freeconference.com. You can use www.audioacrobat.com to record

We recommend doing teleclasses for free at first while getting a sense of what does and doesn't work. Once you feel comfortable, you may charge. Typical fees are anywhere from $19 to $29 per class. You will need to be set up to accept credit cards in order to receive payments for teleclasses. You can use www.paypal.com to collect fees.

reasons to lead a teleclass:
- access to potential clients from the comfort of your home, with no travel time required
- all you need is a phone and a headset
- access to people who can refer you to potential clients
- you build credibility with potential clients
- deepening of relationships with existing clients
- reduced marketing budget (no costs for space or materials)
- get known for being an expert
- talk with people who want to hear what you have to say
- get more participation since shy people can speak up
- an opportunity to test new material and ideas

ways to promote your teleclass:
- send an invitation to every contact on your mailing list
- mention your upcoming teleclass to in-person participants at your workshops
- promote in your newsletter—list the topic description and how to register for the class
- have referral partners and colleagues mention the teleclass to their contact groups and/or list the class in their newsletter
- promote your class on websites that your target market visits
- place a classified listing (free or low cost) in a periodical that your target market frequently reads

how to develop a teleclass:
- brainstorm topics and decide on the content you want to deliver
- design your outline and stages of your talk
- decide who you'd like to invite to your teleclass
- determine how you will market the teleclass
- pick a day and time
- schedule the class

- decide if you'd like to charge for the class
- set up the conference call line
- invite participants (include day and time of talk, plus class description)
- send call-in number and access code to enrolled participants (if charging, send them the financial processing service's link and wait until their payment has been processed)
- send out reminders one or two days before the talk
- practice your talk beforehand

stages of a teleclass curriculum:
- introduction, warmly welcome everyone to your talk
- share your excitement and a personal story about you, and relate that story to your talk
- tell them what to expect from the call, reviewing outline bullet points
- remind them of protocol for the class: pay attention, mute phone when not speaking, put other stuff down
- start your talk, following the outline you created
- do a group share in the middle of the talk to check in around topic content or to see if there are questions
- summarize what you talked about in the call
- thank them for their attention
- allow Q&A, depending on the time remaining
- important: offer invitation to a Health History (ask who is interested and let them know that you will send everyone an email after the call to clarify what the Health History is and how to schedule one)
- send them a special handout, article or other gift after the class
- follow up with the email Health History invitation, including your website, contact information, and a client testimonial or case study
- respond to those who write you

customized programs

If you are already a licensed professional, such as a chiropractor, massage therapist, personal trainer or yoga instructor, you can certainly combine your previous career with health counseling. You can add one or two massages, yoga classes or training sessions to your six-month program and increase the price accordingly. If you are interested in combining health counseling with other practices, consider offering various tiers of service. Create a handout that outlines your different program offerings. Explain your basic six-month health counseling program and list the fee. Then list a medium-priced program that combines health counseling with one extra service each month, such as one massage or private yoga session. Your deluxe program can include two extra services each month. Make sure you give your clients a cost incentive to want to buy the more expensive programs, and let them know that they are getting a discount when they buy more. For example, if your regular program is $150 per month, you can have your medium program cost $225 per month and your deluxe cost $275 per month.

Throughout your career as a health counselor, you can continue to add special offerings to your basic program and see which ones your clients respond to. Other services that graduates have added to their programs with success include monthly food shopping, private monthly cooking classes, Pilates sessions, polarity therapy and fashion consulting. in just three months), or they will want double the support (meeting every week for six months). Again, we recommend that you stick with the standard six-month, every two-week format

At some point, you will come across a client who wants extra support and asks to meet with you once a week. Either they will want to get through the whole program quickly (all 12 sessions for several reasons. First, one week is usually not enough time for a client to try out and fully integrate the recommendations from the previous session. Next, if you do 24 sessions you may find yourself doing extra work by creating new content for the extra sessions. And lastly, you may find yourself giving an unbalanced amount of energy to this one client. Sticking to your every-other-week counseling schedule allows you to keep your own life in balance and be the best counselor possible. You can explain to your client that the six-month program has been proven to be very effective and that they are much more likely to have success in meeting their health goals. However, it is entirely up to you how you work with that person. Experiment and see what works best.

group counseling

Group counseling is a wonderful way for you to expand your practice and reach more people. The group setting creates a community of support and facilitates connections. It is also an opportunity for you to work with people who can't afford your individual program fees. Typical group programs are $75 to $150 per person, per month, depending on where you are with your practice.

If you decide to start a group program, determine your target market. Is it the same target as your regular practice? Do you want to work with lower-income families, kids or men? Once you have that figured out, pick a time and location to best suit the needs of your target market. For example, one of our graduates runs an extremely successful group program for young corporate women at 7:00 am on Wednesday mornings. They meet at her convenient midtown office, have breakfast and participate in group counseling for an hour and a half before work.

Another decision to make regarding your group involves the time frame. Would you like to create a six-month group program or have a rolling-admission group program that always has open admission?

A six-month group program will look something like this:
- you can do individual Health Histories with people interested or hold one orientation for everyone who is interested
- have everyone sign a Program Agreement
- hand out the schedule for the meetings—meeting every other week for six months
- follow the session outlines on the CD-ROM and adapt them appropriately for the group

A rolling-admission group program will look something like this:
- once you have four people who are interested, start your group
- have all participants sign a Program Agreement for six months from the time they enroll
- you can always offer this group program to new clients who can't afford individual programs

A rolling-admission group program will look something like this:

- once you have four people who are interested, start your group
- have all participants sign a Program Agreement for six months from the time they enroll
- you can always offer this group program to new clients who can't afford individual programs
- you can enroll new people into the group at any time, and have each person sign a six-month Program Agreement
- because you'll have new people joining the group at different times, the topics need to be customized to make sense to people who are just starting, as well as people who are in their sixth month of your program
- group size will fluctuate (keep at least four in the group at any given time)
- you can always offer this group program to new clients who can't afford individual programs

An ideal group size is six to 10 people. With this size group, each individual will get enough personalized attention from you and you will be compensated for your time and energy. Generally, your group size should be no less than four and no more than 30 participants. Go about running your group similar to the individual program. You'll have one session every other week and the monthly seminars (you can combine these seminars with the ones you have for your individual clients). You'll use all the same paperwork, give recommendations and provide giveaways at the end of each session. Each session should run anywhere from 90 minutes to two hours, depending on the size of the group. Meet with the group on the same time and day of each week, every two weeks, and have this schedule set before the group begins. Take payments in the same way you do from individuals; have them pay in full, post-dated checks or credit card monthly installments.

Please feel free to customize and enhance with personal touches as you see fit. Get support from your counselor, the OEF and fellow students when creating your group program.

managing a group program

Place the chairs in a circle for smaller groups or in rows of semi-circles for larger groups. Encourage the participants to change seats each time, and to sit next to different people to receive the most value. Be sure that by the beginning of the first session everyone has signed and dated the group Program Agreement.

The group members will feel more comfortable sharing if they trust that their shares will not be judged, and that their confidentiality will be respected. The trust may take some time to develop, but as you remind them that this is a safe space, and that they are welcome to be who they are, without judgment, they will open up and reach their goals more quickly.

Call on people who are quiet and ask them gently to share. Encourage them to speak up, and to remember that when they share, they grow. Everyone in the group should receive individual attention from you at some point during their group program. This may be during their group shares or Q&A, or in individual coaching. You should make sure that all participants feel recognized as individuals. Send personal emails and group emails to check in, let people know you are with them and are truly interested in their growth.

Oftentimes, the more vocal members of the group dominate the conversation. When this happens, lovingly remind them that you are on a schedule and have a lot of important information

completion of your group program: renewal options

It has been my experience that my clients do extremely well during their group program. We cover and they accomplish a lot in a short amount of time. It is also true that many of my clients choose to work with me individually in order to continue this work in greater depth. I am happy to extend this same opportunity to you!

An individual program is perfect for:

- Clients who enjoy a slower and more relaxed pace due to an ultra busy lifestyle and want continued support for another six months.
- Clients who have achieved amazing results in a short amount of time and want to continue with a deeper focus in select areas of concern.
- Clients who would like to work on another goal entirely separate from what they originally started with in the beginning of the group program.
- Clients who simply appreciate the value of my support and services, and who desire a maintenance program.

I've created a few options for graduates of my group program who are interested in continuing to work with me:

- Sign up for an individual program for six months. Your program cost will be a discounted rate of $_____ per month.
- Create a customized program. You and I can agree upon a program that is best for you. Price to be determined.
- Participate in a maintenance program. See me once a month to continue receiving support and working in a comfortable way towards your goals. Price to be determined.

I have enjoyed working with you and welcome the opportunity to continue our work together. If you have any questions, I am happy to help.

Warmly,
Counselor Name
Counselor Contact Info

to cover. Thank them for sharing, and say you'd be happy to talk with them after the group ends. You must be clear with your boundaries. Those who are overly talkative or needy, or who show up late or are disrespectful are not supporting the group dynamic. You should be proactive in handling these situations, but do so with compassion and understanding. At the end of your group program, you can offer individual programs and maintenance programs to the group participants.

corporate clients

You can be successful with corporate clients even if you've never had a corporate job or worn a business suit. Working with corporations is an excellent way to get paid well and to obtain access to a large number of people who could become potential clients. It can also be profitable work for you because companies have a lot of resources.

The first step is to identify the type of corporations where you are interested in working. Is there a particular industry that you find fascinating, have experience with or connections to? Perhaps you have a passion for fashion, and you'd like to work with large department stores or designers. Maybe you have a lot of friends in publishing who might be able to get you into their companies. Or perhaps there is a hedge fund right near where you live that you'd like to become involved with. Spend a little time talking to friends about corporations they know of that might be interested. Also, research on the internet, in the yellow pages and simply drive around your area and take note of companies you may not have noticed before.

Make a list of companies where you would like to offer corporate workshops:

1. _____

2. _____

3. _____

4. _____

5. _____

Make a list of all the people you know in those organizations or in the industry. These people are your best bet for getting connected with the person in the organization in charge of Human Resources and/or corporate wellness programs. Having a pre existing contact will speed up the process of booking a corporate event.

1. _____

2. _____

3. _____

4. _____

5. _____

sample introduction letter to a corporation

Today's date, month and year

Name of Contact
Title of Contact
Name of Corporation
Address of Corporation

Dear (first name of contact):

Thank you for speaking with me about your (corporation, company, center, organization) and how I may be able to support your employees as a health and wellness workshop presenter. I appreciate your consideration.

As you are aware, health benefit costs continue to rise. In the past, employers have tried to lessen these costs by adopting managed care strategies, cost shifting to employees and reducing benefits. These solutions are no longer effectively controlling costs, and are depressing the value of health benefits for employee recruitment and retention. An alternative strategy to contain costs is to improve the health of employees so that less medical care is required. As a health counselor, I provide group workshops that educate your employees on how to improve their health, choose healthier food and take actions towards living a more balanced life.

In this packet I've included a prospectus that details my services and experience as a health counselor, including an overview of my corporate health workshop, the benefits to your organization, my experience and a sample of my writing. Please review the information at your convenience, so that you may have a better understanding of my mission and of the work I do to support corporate employees.

I'm excited about the possibility of contributing my experience to your organization. I will contact you on (date one week later) to answer any questions you may have, and discuss when we can meet in person to plan a workshop. In the meantime, you may reach me at (your number) if you have any questions.

Regards,
Counselor Name
Counselor Contact Info

Once you have identified your contacts, call or email them.

- Tell them that you are a health counselor and corporate workshop presenter.
- Let them know you have a workshop that you present to corporations, educating employees about how to make better food and lifestyle choices, as well as reduce stress in the workplace.
- Ask them who is responsible for corporate wellness workshops or hiring speakers.
- If there is not programming like this in the office, ask for a contact in the HR department.
- Ask your contact to send an email or place a call to say that you will be contacting the company. Your contacts should state that they know you and that you have some valuable information to share about the benefits of health education in the workplace.

Call the names given to you by your contacts.

- Be professional and courteous.
- Introduce yourself, tell them you were referred to them by (contact's name), and that you would like to learn about what they are currently doing to promote health and wellness in the workplace.
- Tell them that you are a certified health counselor, and you present a workshop to a corporation that educates company employees about how to make better choices for food and lifestyle, and how to reduce stress at work.
- Ask them about their company.
- Identify what their needs are and what is important for them, or what may be missing at their company.
- Tell them you would like to learn more about how you can support them in helping their employees to have a happier and healthier workday.
- Remind them of the benefits of these types of programs: reduced absenteeism, lower health care costs and increased productivity, improved community atmosphere and higher employee satisfaction.
- Tell them that you have an information packet that you would like to send them that describes your workshop services. Ask them where you can send it, and let them know you will do this right away and then follow up with them after they have had an opportunity to review the packet.
- Thank them for their time and let them know you are excited to continue learning how you can support them and their organization.

Send your packet (see the CD-ROM for more about materials to include in your packet).

- Use high-quality, professional paper.
- Customize the letter to reflect your knowledge about the company.
- Customize the program offering, putting in specific information you have received about the company.
- Put the packet together: letter, sample program description, bio and newsletter.
- Include your business card in the folder (use a quality, professional folder).
- Use a footer on the documents that includes your contact info.

Follow up, as promised, and request an in-person meeting. Dress professionally for this meeting. Use your charm, be considerate, ask them how they feel you can help their employees. Discuss the different workshops you can offer, and let them know that you can do a one-time workshop or a series. Make a recommendation for which you think would be better, and ask what they think would best suit their needs. Tell them how much you charge for your services. Attempt to schedule a time for your first workshop. It may take several rounds of approval for budget, time and planning before they confirm a date with you. Be patient, but consistent.

Once you have a date in the calendar for the workshop, work with your contact person at the company to ensure that a room has been secured and their employees informed about your workshop. Be sure they are aware of your fee (as negotiated in person).

Prepare for and present your talk. Find a sample outline for a corporate talk on your CD-ROM. You can also use the Sugar Blues or Eating for Energy outlines, adjusting them to make the content pertinent to the work environment.

cold calling

If you do not have corporate contacts, you can use the Internet or business directories to find listings for your favorite companies. Call anyone, ask for the name and number of the person in charge of employee wellness or Human Resources. Get the contact information for that person, and give them a call to introduce yourself and your services.

Cold calling usually takes longer than networking, and not everyone may be as responsive to your request. Even if the company chooses not to work with you, keep them on your mailing list and thank them for their time. They may become interested in the future. Though one opportunity may not happen, there are others that will. Keep moving forward, step by step.

corporate workshop fee

The typical corporate workshop fee is $400 per hour-long session. Multiple sessions are priced at a discounted rate, based on the number of attendees per workshop. This fee includes all materials and handouts. You can price as you feel comfortable, though $300 to $600 per hour is the average range for our graduates.

single workshops

If you've set up a single workshop at a corporation, the goal is to leave with Health Histories scheduled and with the participants feeling that they benefited from your presentation. You want the corporation to speak highly of you, to refer you to other corporations, and potentially invite you back for another workshop or a series of workshops.

workshop series

When pitching your services to a corporation, you might want to offer three workshops—one a month for 3 months—or you may want to offer a six-month program with 12 different workshops. Let the person you are speaking with know that you can do single workshops or a series. Explain that if they get a series, their employees will experience greater benefits and the company will save money.

Dear Employer,

If you are concerned about your employees' long-term health and have noticed the connection between wellness and productivity, we invite you to participate in the [your company name] Wellness Series.

Preventable diseases cost businesses thousands of dollars a year. Recent research shows that over 50% of absenteeism at the workplace can be attributed to stress and stress-related illnesses. According to the Director of Health Care Management at Ford Motors, weight-related expenses alone are costing employers approximately $12 billion per year. A 2003 Chrysler Corporation study showed that employees with poor eating habits generated 41% more healthcase claim costs than those with good eating habits (Missouri Western State College, Krueger, Wampler, Adams, 2003).

Across the country, companies are beginning to take notice of the startling connections between employee wellness and fiscal responsibility, and look for better answers. Employee wellness programs not only boost morale, but also make significant, measurable differences in healthcare spending. Studies have shown that employee wellness programs help companies reduce their healthcare costs an average of $3.72 for each dollar invested!

[Your company name] is proud to present its Wellness Series, comprised of 12 programs designed to inspire employees to take significant, preventative steps for their long-term health and wellness. The Wellness Series is accessible to a wide range of people, and addresses the most common current health issues, including low energy, stress, weight loss, high blood pressure and cholesterol, and how to incorporate healthy lifestyle choices into busy schedules.

Programs in the series run 60 to 90 minutes, and trainers are highly interactive with the audience, incorporating exercises, visual aids, handouts and other media. A teleclass format is also available.

The Wellness Series gives employees the skills to take control of their wellness by deepening their knowledge of the effect of nutrition and lifestyle changes on their health. The series is excellent training to help employees make the best choices to sustain their vitality and productivity for years to come.

Thank you for your interest in [your company name] Wellness Series. This packet contains detailed information about our 12-program series, my biography and testimonials from recent clients. Please feel free to contact me for more information or to schedule a workshop in the coming months.

Sincerely,
Counselor Name
Counselor Contact Info

courtesy of Cheryl Mirabella

phone counseling

Health counseling is just as effective when done over the phone as it is in person. Phone counseling is a great way to expand your practice, and to work from the comfort of your home. It is perfect for clients who are busy, want the convenience of calling from home or the office, travel frequently for business or pleasure, want to reduce commuting time, live outside your area or are single and/or working parents who need to be home during evening hours.

Phone counseling works well for counselors who don't have an office space, want to work from home but don't want clients there, like to travel or don't want to be encumbered with an in-person client schedule. If you like to talk on the phone and enjoy the flexibility of being able to do your sessions from anywhere, phone counseling may be a great fit for you.

If you know you want to do phone counseling, be sure to mention it in your marketing materials. Simply call or email potential clients, let them know about this new work you are doing and invite them to do a Health History with you over the phone. Let them know what to expect: that you will email them the Health History, that they can fill it out and send it back or that you'll fill it out together over the phone. Send them a reminder email or give them a quick phone call the day before, suggesting they put aside an hour of time in a quiet and comfortable space for your call. Consider asking them to have a glass of water or cup of tea handy.

Have your clients call you, just as if they were coming to you for an in-person session. This has them take responsibility for their session and also saves you the phone bill.

When they have called in, ask them a question to create relatedness and connection. Maybe you'll ask how their day was, or something that is new and good. Check in that they are in a comfortable, quiet and private space. Proceed to go over the Health History as you would in person, asking them questions, listening and avoiding giving advice.

After they've agreed to work with you, take their credit card number over the phone to hold their first official session of their program. Even if you don't have a credit card merchant account, it has them take you seriously. If you do have a merchant account (ability to accept credit cards), bill them immediately for the first month. Tell them you will need to have post-dated checks (if they are paying in this way) and the signed Program Agreement at least 24 hours before their first session. Schedule all 12 sessions with them while you have them on the phone. Ask them to get their scheduler and put in the dates.

After you get off the phone, email them the Program Agreement, welcome letter and reminder of when their sessions begin. Encourage them to fax or mail the forms back as soon as they can.

A six-month program over the phone works almost identically to an in-person program. You meet once every two weeks for an hour, listen to your clients, provide recommendations and follow the same structure for your sessions that you would in person. At the end of each session, send them a quick email telling them how great the call went and give them your notes. Email them any handouts you would have given them at an in-person session. Be sure to email them shortly after the call. Print the notes out for your reference.

We recommend that you ship them all their giveaways in two separate installments, one after they sign up for your program and one halfway through. This makes less work for you because you don't have to go to the post office each week, and it also makes your clients feel special because everyone loves getting gifts in the mail. After they sign and fax or mail you the Program Agreement, mail them their first giveaway package, including their binder for the handouts and recipes that you will email them after each session. You'll also want to include one giveaway for each session through the third month—six giveaways total. Be sure to make a note of which ones you sent so you know what to send in the second package.

Here are some phone counseling tips:

- Invest in a hands-free headset with mute facility.
- If possible, meet your client in person at least once during your six-month program.
- If you cannot meet in person, exchange photos over email or via snail mail.
- Start on time and end on time.
- Give the client a warm welcome and check in at the beginning of the session.
- Remind them to put down any other things they may be doing, and to find a private, quiet and comfortable space.
- Begin session with a simple breathing exercise or grounding exercise to slow their pace from the day and to be present with you.
- Do not multi-task while on the phone.
- Be conscious of the tone of your voice, and don't speak too quickly
- Make sure the client knows you are listening.
- Ask questions, be interested.
- Don't be afraid of silences.
- Take notes.
- Direct them as to which mailed giveaway corresponds with which session.
- Email or send them a copy of the session notes page, along with the action steps you outlined, once you complete the session.
- For consistency, if you send follow-up emails to check in with the clients, you should do so regularly and at the same time interval.
- Follow up at the next session as to whether they tried the recommendations.

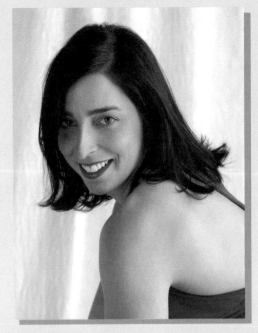

For six years I was a manager of the Juvenile Diabetes Foundation International. For as long as I could remember I had a lingering feeling that I could be doing more with my life. It didn't help that I was always stressed out—working the corporate job with long hours, long commutes and suffering from digestive trouble.

When I nearly lost my life in an accident, I realized that I was alive for a purpose, so I began exploring what that was. Six months later I enrolled at Integrative Nutrition. Within two months I had several clients. Three months after graduation I quit my day job and started my own business as a certified health counselor.

My clients are super busy, overworked, stressed-out business owners and executives. They struggle with how to be healthy, have a family life and have a social life. Once

Jenn Edden
Syosset, NY
jennedden@yahoo.com
2004 Graduate

they see that they are choosing unhealthy foods because of their stressful lifestyles, and not because they lack willpower, they drop the "diet mentality" and begin to put better fuel in their bodies.

With my support, my clients see concrete results. They lose weight and lower their blood pressure and cholesterol. They manage their time and their stress much better. Most importantly, they stop being so hard on themselves. They are so used to functioning in a world where they are constantly being evaluated. Helping my clients redefine success is a major part of their healing process.

Getting support from my colleagues has been essential to my success. It is imperative to have one or two friends as your cheerleaders to run your ideas by, share what you are up to, ask for help, and get feedback and support. Also, creating simple systems for my business has helped me stay organized. I have a new client checklist, which includes a reminder to input client contact information into my computer, add client birthdays to my calendar, create a client folder with handouts and include clients on my monthly newsletter distribution list. In addition, I always make extra copies of handouts and buy extra giveaways, so I don't have to do the work every time I get a new client. Friday is my day to organize and plan for the week ahead so I can start my week off on the right foot, with time allotted for seeing clients, marketing my business and, most importantly, some down time for me!

I feel so privileged to be out there making a real difference in peoples' lives. I'm excited to be branching out into the corporate speaking arena, and I just gave my first paid talk to 15 employees. I was recently a guest on a talk radio show, The Wizard of Is (1240AM), where I was introduced as a board certified health counselor and was able to take calls from listeners. It felt great to be on the radio, and I know I'd even like to break into television at some point. I constantly remind myself that that this is my life, not a dress rehearsal!

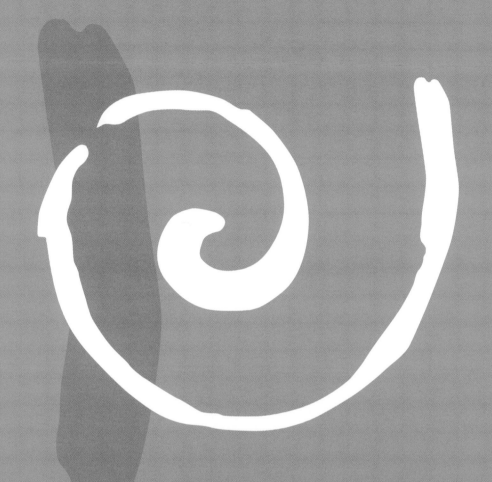

chapter seven

If you light a lamp for somebody,
it will also brighten your path.

Buddhist saying

counseling clients

Y

ou are beginning to know what it feels like to be a health counselor. You are most likely discovering that health counseling is a highly rewarding undertaking and a lot more interesting than watching television or working at your computer. The core of our work as health counselors is to support our clients on their journey to health and wellness. We are a source of loving encouragement, we share helpful tips and we help them move forward with their goals. It is a highly rewarding undertaking.

In your work with clients, you are going to have some who are gems and some who are more difficult. In this chapter we provide you with some ideas on how to work successfully with all your clients, and what to do if and when you have clients who are difficult or who have complex health concerns that demand the services of a medical professional.

tips for successful client-counselor relationships

increase foods that support health

If you can get your clients to eat more greens, vegetables, whole grains, sweet vegetables and healthy fats and proteins, you will dramatically change their lives. The food we eat makes our blood and our cells, and creates our thoughts. By supporting your clients to increase healthy foods, they will see and feel the changes in themselves. Unhealthy foods will get crowded out, and your clients will be motivated to progress even further.

reduce foods that don't support health

As you know, most health conditions will improve with the reduction of meat, milk, sugar, caffeine and artificial/chemicalized junk food. Work slowly to add healthier options into you clients' diets, so that over time they can reduce foods that don't support health and energy.

start with secondary food, then incorporate primary food

Many health counselors have their food figured out. They know what foods work for them, and how to eat to get the most energy. Sometimes they automatically think everyone else has this figured out as well. These counselors often jump right into primary food issues with their clients, skipping over the incremental education around secondary food. This is not an effective strategy. If you want your clients to experience change and increased health, the best thing you can do is work with them on secondary food first. Get them eating leafy greens, whole grains, high-quality protein and home-cooked food. Once they have these foods as part of their regular diet, you can begin to look at the primary food issues that are out of balance and need change. Without changing the food that people eat first, it is difficult to change their lifestyle choices.

love up your clients

Offer unending encouragement and support. Compliment them on their progress often. Send them a card or letter in the mail acknowledging how far they have come. Remember details about their lives, such as pets' and family members' names. Let them know you are happy to be working with them.

listen

Provide your clients with a safe space to talk and be heard. When you are present with clients and actively listen, you will find that your intuition will guide you during your session. Oftentimes, the client just wants to talk. You don't have to solve their problems. By simply having someone who listens, your client will figure out the answers to their issues.

define client goals

When you begin a health counseling program, it is important to have the client fill out the Welcome Handout, where they clearly define their goals for the program. Clients must first be aware of their present situation and define what they would like to accomplish. It is also valuable to continually check in with the client around their progress towards goals. You can create new goals or redefine existing goals as their program continues.

follow session outlines

We provide you with outlines for each of your sessions (1 through 12) on the CD-ROM. You do not need to follow them word for word, but the outlines provide direction for you and the client. Review the outline for each client session before the session begins.

focus on the positives

Always start your sessions by asking the client what is new and good. Often, people tend to focus only on what is not going well. As you help clients focus on what they are doing that is positive and what is good in their lives, they create a space for more good to enter.

handouts and giveaways

Provide the client with handouts and giveaways (food samples, CDs, books, self-care items) at each session. You can follow the guidelines set up in the session outlines on the CD-ROM. Feel free to add your own touches.

two or three recommendations per session

End your sessions with two or three simple recommendations that the client can work on until you meet for your next session. Remember, it is important to not overwhelm the client with too much work, and you should always go at a pace that's comfortable for the client.

ask questions

Ask clients questions to get them thinking. You don't need to come up with all the answers to your clients' problems. They know more about their lives than you do. With the appropriate questions, they will figure out so much on their own. You can ask, "Why?", "What?", "How is that working for you?", "What do you think you should do?", "What do you think you should eat?", "Who can you turn to for more support?" Let the client respond and come up with their own conclusions.

help your client get support

Encourage your clients to get support outside of your sessions from sources such as family, friends, community, spiritual groups and other groups that encourage connection and community.

personalize the program

If you have expertise in other areas related to health, such as yoga, Pilates or massage, you can incorporate these into your program. Chances are, if there is something that you enjoy doing that has helped you with your own health and happiness, your clients could benefit from it as well. Add your personal touch and complement the program with topics specific to each client and their goals.

keep track of client progress

Keep track of your clients' progress between each session on the Client Progress Form. Remind your clients of what they are accomplishing while working with you.

responsibility

Let the clients take ownership of their health, have them commit and be willing to do the work.

create a partnership

Clients are accustomed to relating to hired professionals as experts or authority figures. Collaboration works best when there are no traditional roles. Get out of the need to claim all the credit or have all the answers.

be a compassionate guide

You don't need to tell your clients everything they should do. Ask them what they want you to do or not to do in the program. You are not healing them, they're healing themselves. Be honored to be a part of the process. You actually help the client more when you are less attached to getting results. When you are attached to outcome, you can get tense and stop breathing as deeply. Take deep breaths often during sessions to release attachment.

dedication

Put your focus on the client, on what the client wants and on ways to help them achieve it. Be committed to clients' goals, outcomes, growth, learning, experimentation, integrity, discovery and evolution. Try offering new food options and new ideas, and help them make your suggestions a priority. Make sure they know they need to be dedicated. You will support them and hold them accountable, but they need to be motivated to do the work.

be gentle but demanding

Being too soft or nice doesn't do clients justice. Not confronting an issue because it makes you uncomfortable is unfair to the client.

respect differences

Remember your client is not you. Meet your client where they are. Do not impose your views on what is nutritionally right. You are probably highly advanced; you have been interested in nutrition for quite some time. Not everyone is as in tune with their diet as you are. Let the client set a pace that is comfortable for them. You can give them an extra push, but you want to set them up for success. Go slowly and give them recommendations you know they will follow.

courtesy

Insist that you are both on time, prepared for sessions and show up feeling 100%. Have the client pay on time, don't reschedule appointments, clarify your rescheduling protocol for yourself and go over your policies with the client, especially if they miss or arrive late to a session.

client retention

There are two aspects to client retention. One is keeping your clients satisfied with the six-month program so they don't want to withdraw. The other is re-signing clients for another six months or a maintenance program when their first program is up.

You want each and every one of your clients to be a raving fan of you and your program. You want your clients to be so thrilled about working with you that they tell everyone they know about you, and maybe even sign up with you for a second six-month program. And the happier your clients are with you, the more enjoyable it will be for you to work with them.

The best way to create raving fans is to support your clients on achieving the goals they set forth in the beginning of their program. Be in constant communication about what their goals are and how you can support them to attain these aspirations.

To keep your clients happy, it is extremely important that you maintain a high level of professionalism: that you are on time, prepared, do what you say you are going to do, consistently send them notes after each session and reminders before each session. You do not want to let your clients down in any way. They depend on you to be their support system, and even if you are a day late in doing something that you promised you would do (such as email an article or give them the address to a yoga studio), they will take it to mean that they were not a priority.

Like we said before, you must get the payment from your clients at the beginning of their program. Once the money is out of the way, in their minds it has already been paid for. If they have to write you a new check every month or pay you in cash every month, they may question the purchase each time. Getting payment up-front is crucial to retaining clients.

Make sure your clients feel that their program is individualized. Provide giveaways that relate to what you've talked about in your sessions. Make recommendations based on their individual circumstances. Send clients' notes in the mail letting them know how well they are doing. You may also want to incorporate personalized welcome letters or birthday cards. When it comes time to give them the giveaway at the end of each session, let them know how it will be helpful for them, considering what they are going through. Even if it's a tongue scraper and they have not talked about their dental health, let them know that using a tongue scraper is a great way to reduce cravings or increase the satisfaction of kissing. They will appreciate your thoughtfulness. These little extra touches do not take a lot of your time and will add tremendously to customer satisfaction.

Take into account that the higher your customer's satisfaction is, the more enjoyable your job will become. If your clients are happy to see you, tell you about how much they love working with you and also spread the word to others, your confidence will increase, as will the size of your business and your personal fulfillment.

re-signing clients

As you come to the end of a six-month program, you can offer your client the opportunity to work with you for six more months. It's best to offer this to clients who you truly enjoy working with and whom you think would benefit from more of your support. It might feel scary to ask clients to keep seeing you, but what do you have to lose? Simply let them know that you are interested and available for further support. Chances are they are wondering how they are going to manage without seeing you anymore! A second six-month program can be enormously significant for clients. They already have a trusting relationship with you, and they are healthier and more clear thinking than they were six months earlier. In their second program they are able to work very deeply on creating a life they love.

To re-sign clients, at the end of session 10 or 11, mention to them that you have a special deal for people who sign up a second time. Let them know that however far they came in your work together, they will continue to grow and thrive even more over the next six months. This gives them some time to think about what they want their life to look like after their program ends.

You can also offer them a maintenance program, seeing them once a month for six months or every other week for three months. This lower cost, lower commitment arrangement can appeal to clients who crave more support but don't have the time or resources to do another six-month program. If your client is having difficulty deciding what's best for them, use your closing deal skills to walk them through the process. If they decide to work with you again, re-sign the appropriate Program Agreement, get their payment, set up their new appointments and congratulate them on making such a powerful commitment to themselves and their health.

ideal clients

As we discussed in Chapter 4, in the beginning of your career as a health counselor, you will take on different types of clients—various ages, income levels, and both men and women. Working with a variety of people will help you discover which types of clients you enjoy most. It will soon become clear which clients energize and inspire you. It is these people whom you should declare your ideal clients and build your target market strategy around.

The clearer you are about the clients you want to work with, the easier it will be for you to find them and for them to find you. Believe us; it is possible to have a thriving part-time or full-time practice working with clients who you truly enjoy. You need not suffer working with clients who make your life miserable simply for the paycheck or for experience. We encourage you to only take on clients you find pleasure in working with.

my ideal client

In order to attract your ideal client, first identify what that client would be like. Use this chart to get clear about the characteristics and personality traits that your client must have, preferably has, preferably does not have and must not have. If you already have one ideal client, you can use that person's qualities as a guide.

Must Have	Preferably Has	Preferably Does Not Have	Must Not Have

Take a moment to look at your ideal client chart every day. As you become more mindful of exactly who you are looking for, you will notice that type of person showing up more frequently in your life.

difficult clients

Working with clients who are difficult will drain your energy and stifle the progress of your practice. Your program is an intimate relationship that is shared for six months. Being in that relationship with even one client who creates complications can ruin your exhilaration and motivation around being a health counselor.

Try to identify potentially difficult clients during the Health History and do not sign them up for your program. Here are some red flags for the types of clients you may not want to work with:

- Those who don't show up or come late and make excuses. If they do this from the beginning, they will most likely continue through the entire program.
- People who complain over every detail of the program or the Program Agreement. An ideal client is ready and willing to sign up and enjoy your program, but a difficult client has many hesitations.
- People who challenge you and question your abilities. If someone isn't sure they want to work with you, it means probably they will not be successful in your program.
- Individuals who try to negotiate fees. People who take an inch will often try to take a mile down the road.
- People who don't do the work, resist your guidance, make excuses or lie.
- Any people who, for whatever reason, get on your nerves so dramatically that it is difficult to be around them. Some people will not be a good fit for you. Don't resist the obvious. Let them walk out the door and save yourself the agony.

If someone who fits this description comes to a Health History, simply complete the Health History and thank them for coming. Escort them out without explaining your program or the fees. If they ask you about it, you can honestly say that you don't think the two of you would make a good fit working together. You don't need to go into detail about why, just politely send them on their way.

If you already have difficult clients, it is best to discontinue your work with them. You can explain to them that your skill set is not suited to match their specific needs. Let them know you can provide a referral to another practitioner who is better suited to help them reach their goals. You can refund their money, prorated for the number of months you worked together, or give them back their post-dated checks. Let them go, and focus your energy on getting more ideal clients.

preventing no-shows

The absolute best way to prevent no-shows at scheduled sessions is to have your clients pay up-front and to be clear from the beginning about your lateness and attendance policies. If you do not get paid, either in full with post-dated checks or with a credit card number up-front, you are sending a message to your clients that they do not have to be committed. Let them know that if they don't give you 24-hour notice for a cancellation they cannot make up the session.

You may also want to send out a reminder email or phone call the day before each session. Confirm the time and place of your appointment, and let them know that you look forward to seeing them.

when a client wants to withdraw

There are a few reasons why clients may want to withdraw from your program. The most common grounds are fear, not achieving their expected results, thinking they already know everything and financial issues.

In most cases, this will happen halfway through your six-month program. If and when this happens, share with your client that this is common. Tell them that many people go through this at the halfway point. You can gently remind them that they signed a Program Agreement, which is legally binding. Remind them how far they have come. Explain why the program is six months long—to build long-term habits. Give them the space to express their concerns. Ask them if there is anything that they would like to see happen moving forward. You can mention a few things that you see them accomplishing over the next three months, and tell them you look forward to supporting them in making those changes. Most people who contemplate withdrawing from your program are basking for more support in a roundabout way.

In special circumstances, you may want to let your client withdraw. If they lost their jobs and genuinely cannot afford it, if they were diagnosed with a serious illness or if they are extremely difficult clients, it may be in your best interest to discontinue the program and refund them the money for sessions that have not yet occurred. To prevent withdrawals, be in constant communication with your clients about their goals and what they are looking for from your work together.

working with children

Working with young people can be extremely rewarding. Getting five-year-olds to eat kale on a regular basis is an incredible accomplishment because their lives will turn out completely differently than if they were just eating McDonald's and Doritos.

If you enjoy the company of children and you would like to incorporate them into your client base, go for it! You can work with them just as you would with any other client—meeting twice a month for six months. See your CD-ROM for a special Health History you can use with children.

Don't underestimate children. They are often more open to change and new foods than adults give them credit for. Because they have not been alive as long, children do not have as many habits built up as adults do. They are often more in touch with their bodies and surroundings than adults. With the right support, they have strong instincts about how to get themselves well.

Spend a good amount of time at the start of your program building rapport and connection. This is critical because it makes your child client feel safe enough to open up to you. Ask great questions, lead them gently and allow them to trust you. Show them you understand their situation. Treat them with respect. Be encouraging. Make them feel special and heard.

Children are spontaneous. You may need to shorten your sessions or incorporate movement and stretch breaks to keep their attention and focus. You don't want their time with you to feel too serious.

Ways to add fun to your sessions with children:

- Lead them on a kid-friendly health food store tour.
- Let them come up with their own recommendations.
- Make kid-friendly food together, such as ice pops or "ants on a log."
- Meet somewhere unexpected such as a playground or on pillows on your office floor.
- Bring in food, giveaways and other props for them to touch, look at, taste and discover.
- Give them stickers and different colored pens to use in their food journal and notebook.

Keep in mind that it takes children three tries to like a new food. The first time it is usually too new, the second time they still don't like it, but by the third try their taste buds usually come around. So be patient.

Depending on the age of your client, the parent will play a major role in the program. In some cases a parent may sit in on sessions. During the Health History determine how involved the parents of your child clients will be, and make sure everyone is on the same page. When working with children ages 12 and under, here are some tips on how to have the parents involved:

- Give parents all handouts so that they understand the work their child is doing with you.
- Provide the parents with recipes and bring them along on the health food store tour so they become aware of how to incorporate healthier foods into the household.

Some graduates who work with children have every other session with the parent and every other session with the child. This way they get to work with the parent around how to balance their life while raising a child. They teach the parent cooking techniques, and support the parent in being a healthy example. In the sessions with the child, the counselor introduces healthy snack foods and talks about the food-mood connection and primary food.

teenage clients

Teenagers usually respond very well to working with health counselors. Most seek adults who they can confide in and look up to. If you are interested in working with teenagers, you can begin by offering workshops at high schools and teen camps. If your goal is to sign up clients for a six-month program, we recommend you invite the parents to the workshops as well because they are the ones who are going to pay for and probably drive the teenager to see you. You want to show the parents your professionalism and the potential health benefits for their child. Having parental support and encouragement will greatly increase your teen clients' satisfaction and success in your program.

Teens react well to being granted greater responsibility and being treated like adults, so the parents of your teenage clients need not be closely involved in the six-month program. When signing the Program Agreement, make it clear that your sessions will be between you and the teenager only. You can invite the parent to attend the monthly seminars as a guest of your teenage client.

If your teenage client shares with you information that could affect their safety or others, it is imperative that you support your client in telling their parents. Examples of this are drug use, suicidal comments, violent tendencies and eating disorders. If your client refuses to tell their parents, you must tell them yourself. Telling parents the truth will help your clients overcome their struggles.

health counseling parameters

Health counselors do not heal anyone. Clients do the work and are responsible for their own life and health. We are their "guide on the side."

It is important not to work with clients who have major health concerns or who are taking multiple prescription drugs. Their concerns are often too complex, and are best supported through other means.

When working with clients who have minor health concerns, use the reference guides we gave you to look up their ailments. *The Complete Guide to Nutritional Healing* and *Healing with Whole Foods* are two excellent sources of information. You can look up conditions from migraine headaches to acid reflux, from dandruff to candida. These books will give dietary suggestions to help people overcome certain health concerns. You can share these tools with your clients by photocopying the pages that relate to their specific conditions. Also, if you have clients who take one or two medications, use the Physicians Desk Reference (PDR) to investigate possible side effects and contraindications (food or otherwise) associated with medications.

You should never tell a client to stop taking medications, or to stop seeing their doctor or psychiatrist. Nor should you ever encourage clients to make radical life changes (quitting a job, leaving a relationship, moving out of town). Clients will come up with their own solutions to their problems, and when they do so you can support them with the decisions they make. However, the client is in charge of their life, and they are ultimately responsible for the outcomes of their decisions. In order to protect yourself against any possible liability, be sure to always have your clients fill out the Program Agreement and explain to them that they are responsible for their own decisions.

when to refer clients

As a new health counselor, you should seek out clients who are in good overall health. Clients should not be on multiple medications. They should not have seriously advanced, chronic, critical or complex health conditions, such as cancer, degenerative illnesses or life-threatening eating disorders. Some chronic conditions—such as autoimmune disorders like diabetes, thyroid issues and metabolic syndromes—are acceptable. However, in these cases the client should also be under the care of a medical practitioner. We recommend the client alert their practitioner that they are in your program. This way, you can help support the efforts and recommendations of the medical care provider. If you are unsure about working with any particular client, you should seek the advice of your counselor or a trusted healthcare professional, and err on the side of caution.

Sometimes clients may not reveal this information until they are already into the program with you. In this case it is imperative that the clients already be working with a healthcare professional and that the professional knows the client is working with you. If the client has cancer, a life-threatening illness or a serious chronic condition and refuses to work with a medical care professional, we strongly urge you to stop working with that client to protect both parties involved. You can refer these clients to a medical doctor, osteopath, naturopath or nurse practitioner. Health counseling is not a substitute for seeing a medical professional.

It is helpful for beginning health counselors to keep certain distinctions in mind in order to determine if a client needs additional support from a mental health professional. Developing active listening is the best way to be aware of whether or not you should refer your client to another professional to check for underlying complex medical or emotional issues.

Listen to your intuition. If you think you might be in over your head, you most likely are. Set and trust your boundaries. Don't let your desire to be helpful or your fear of rejecting someone allow you to be drawn into an inappropriate situation. Depending on the extent of your client's condition, you may still be able to work with the client while they are seeking medical or mental health treatment.

If your client shows signs of depression, mania, mental instability or suicidal tendencies, you should refer them immediately to a mental health professional.

signs of depression:
- decreased energy, fatigue
- feelings of hopelessness, pessimism
- persistent sad, anxious or "empty" mood
- feelings of guilt, worthlessness, helplessness
- thoughts of death or suicide, suicide attempts
- appetite and/or weight loss, overeating, weight gain
- insomnia, early morning awakening or oversleeping
- difficulty concentrating, remembering, making decisions
- loss of interest in pleasure or hobbies that were once enjoyable, including sex

signs of mania:
- poor judgment
- racing thoughts
- increased talking
- suicidal thoughts
- grandiose notions
- unusual irritability
- increased sexual desire
- decreased need for sleep
- markedly increased energy
- inappropriate social behavior
- abnormal or excessive elation

signs of mental instability:
- Is the client out of touch with reality, fixated on events of the past?
- Are they emotionally unable to cope or to follow through on basic strategies, excessively anxious, emotional or angry?
- Do they suffer from the result of a recent trauma, domestic violence or grief/loss?
- Is there a substance abuse issue or other serious addiction involved?

A client's reference to suicidal thoughts or tendencies should be taken very seriously. Handle them in the following ways:

- When talking about thoughts of suicide with a client, do not swear to secrecy.
- Ask the client if they are currently having thoughts of suicide or have a suicide plan. Be aware that the more detailed the plan and the greater the access to the means to carry out the plan, the greater the risk of suicide.
- Ask them if they are working with a mental health professional. If they are not, have them contact their doctor or the suicide hotline in your area to get a referral. They can also go to the local hospital.
- Have them make a plan to meet with someone either on the spot or within the next few hours. (If there will be an interval of time before they will be meeting with the person, ask them to agree with you to not take any actions to hurt themselves at least until they meet with the professional. Help them to identify and call a support person that can come and be with them until their appointment in order to help them stay safe and reduce feelings of isolation.)
- If the client is a minor, talk to their parent or guardian about how to keep the client safe. Remind parents that if alcohol or drug use is involved, suicide risk is increased.

Who to refer depressed and suicidal clients to:
- doctor
- therapist
- psychiatrist
- psychologist
- rehab program
- licensed social worker
- mental health counselor

Making a professional link with a mental health professional is a good idea. You can refer clients to them if need be, and they can act as a resource on matters related to mental health.

additional issues to consider for referrals
Child Abuse and Maltreatment is defined as:
- sexual abuse
- malnourishment
- use of drugs or alcohol
- extreme emotional abuse
- improper/inadequate supervision
- substantial risk for physical injury
- physical abuse, injury or excessive corporal punishment
- inadequate shelter, clothing, education, medical or surgical care

In the event that you witness or it is revealed to you that a minor is being abused or neglected in some way, we advise that a report be made to the child welfare agency or hotline in your area. The reporting phone number is usually printed in the front of your phone book or listed under your local department of social services.

If it is an emergency situation, the police should be called.

If the person who revealed the instance of child abuse to you is the direct witness, encourage the witness to call and make a report. However, if you believe a child is truly in danger, we suggest you make the call. If you are not in a profession in which you are legally mandated to report these issues, you may do so anonymously.

If a client reveals that they were the victim of a relatively recent crime, such as rape or domestic violence, encourage them to report the incident to the local police department. In addition, the client should be encouraged to meet with a therapist or visit an intervention agency that deals with the post-traumatic issues of such events.

The above is also relevant in cases where the incident occurred in the not-so-recent past. If a client still feels threatened by the perpetrator of a past crime at the present time, they should be encouraged to seek legal support or work with an appropriate intervention agency.

fraud factor

At this point some of you still might not be seeing clients. Maybe you aren't even telling people that you are a health counselor. For one reason or another you feel you are not equipped to counsel the public. Maybe you are waiting until you graduate, until you've read all the books and heard from all the visiting teachers or until your own health is "perfect." You are thinking, "Who am I to tell other people what to do around their health?" You feel like a fraud when you label yourself a professional health counselor. This is what we call the Fraud Factor.

List all the reasons why you feel unequipped to counsel the public:

1. _____

2. _____

3. _____

4. _____

5. _____

6. _____

7. _____

8. _____

Where do these beliefs come from?

1. _____

2. _____

3. _____

4. _____

5. _____

How can you let go of these self-limitations and create new thought patterns centered on your incredible skill and intuition as a health counselor?

_____

_____

_____

_____

_____

_____

_____

_____

We are here to tell you that you are not a fraud. You already know more about health than most of the people on this planet. Your knowledge, along with the tools we teach you, is enough to help people increase their health and happiness. You do not need to be 100% healthy and perfect to be a health counselor. All you need is to be able to listen, ask questions, give recommendations and use the resources you have available to you.

This is the time to start seeing clients! Identify what is keeping you from getting out there and sharing what you know and who you are. Your busy schedule? Low self-esteem? Thinking you don't know enough about nutrition? Use your counselor and use the school to help you overcome these obstacles. This is the year when you will have the most support. This is the year to begin. You have something very valuable to share with people, so get out there!

When I started classes at Integrative Nutrition, I did not intend to start a business. I planned to use this education in the doctors' office where I work as a cardiac nurse. But when a coworker found out what I was doing, she asked me if I would work with her. Before I knew it, I was graduating with ten clients and my own part-time business.

Before coming to the school, I lived my life in search of losing the last ten pounds. As a marathon runner and figure skater who is prone to high cholesterol, I could never find any dietary advice that fit with my athletic training. While attending the school, I figured out exactly how to eat for my body and lifestyle. Now I don't care what my weight is because I feel so good.

In my business, I have three different target markets: health professionals, people with high cholesterol and athletes. I work with stressed-out healthcare workers because I was one of them before coming to Integrative Nutrition. I was a burnt-out, frustrated nurse, and now I am a healthy, happy health counselor who looks forward

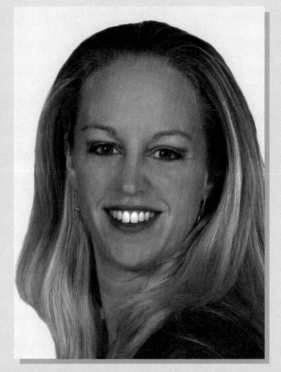

Kelley Dobbins
Watertown, CT
kelsice@aol.com
2005 Graduate

to the work I do every day. I help my colleagues in healthcare understand that they need to prioritize their own health and well-being so they can be in a better position to take care of others. This is something that we never learned in nursing school, and I believe it is one of the main reasons for the nursing shortage today. In addition to my private clients, I work with patients in the doctors' office to reduce their dependency on drugs for lowering their cholesterol levels. I also enjoy working with athletes to increase their performance through nutrition and creative visualization. I teach them to enjoy their training and development as much as the ultimate outcome, a pivotal shift I made during my year in school.

Becoming a health counselor has changed my life. Before Integrative Nutrition, I was always invisible and afraid of failure. I never wanted to make a mistake, and now I embrace mistakes as a way to learn. I now know whatever my dream, I can make it happen. Working with clients to give them the tools to make healthy food choices, not obsess over what they eat, and take good care of themselves is the best job in the world. In nursing there is no time to listen, but in health counseling I know the best tool I have is my listening skills.

Nurses are taught to stay quiet in the background. We let the doctors do the talking and make important decisions. This completely changed for me while in school. I learned to speak up, find my voice and recognize that what I have to say is incredibly valuable. I never thought I'd have my own business and speak in front of groups. I am even writing a book with one of the doctors on cholesterol management, something that I would not have been able to do without the confidence I developed while at the school. If I can do this, anyone can do it!

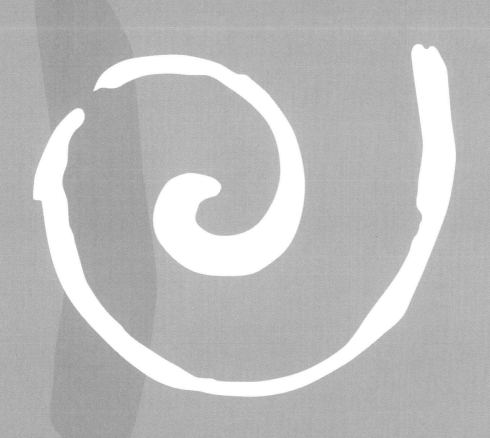

chapter eight

It is common sense to take a method and try it.
If it fails, admit it frankly and try another.
But above all, try something.

Franklin D. Roosevelt

smart marketing

arketing is any method of attracting and retaining customers. It is not just your website, flyers and advertisements. It goes far beyond the tools laid forth in this chapter and this book. All of your business activity becomes part of your marketing effort, including the way you set up your office, how you greet strangers, the writing of your newsletter and the clothes you put on each morning.

The key to successful marketing is discovering what works for you and the personality of your unique business. Some graduates get 90% of their clients from workshops. Other graduates never lead workshops and get all their clients from referral systems with other health professionals. A number of graduates make a constant effort to get into the press and advertise frequently in holistic magazines. There is no one-size-fits-all rule when it comes to marketing. Explore the different resources available and choose what feels right to you, and what produces the most results.

marketing review

In Chapter 4 we introduced some of the core methods of getting clients. Here is that list again.

- website
- press kit
- brochures
- newsletter
- workshops
- health fairs
- networking
- business cards

Which of these techniques have you already tried?

_____

_____

What has been most effective for you so far?

_____

_____

_____

_____

What current marketing materials do you use regularly?

_____

_____

_____

Do your materials reflect your target market and are they in alignment with your mission statement?

_____

_____

_____

_____

What methods would you like to add to your marketing repertoire?

_____

_____

_____

_____

barriers to success

- You can't decide where to begin—Marketing your business seems like an overwhelming project. There are too many considerations and choices. You want to make sure you do it all perfectly, so you worry about how to best spend your time. Struck by "analysis paralysis," you start and stop, sit and stew, or just do nothing.
- You aren't sure how to put the pieces together—You know you should be leading workshops, writing a newsletter and doing Health Histories, but you think that you should finish your brochure or design your logo or read one more nutrition book first. You don't have a system, a program or a plan.
- You can't stay motivated—With no boss holding you accountable, it's easy to procrastinate around marketing. If you don't see immediate results, you can get discouraged and lose motivation. It's difficult to not take it personally when someone doesn't sign up for your program.

If you have ever had any of these thoughts or if you are having them now, you are not alone. People who market service businesses rarely fail due to lack of information about effective sales and marketing techniques. They fail because they don't use the information that is right at their fingertips. Use the techniques laid out in this book, what we teach in class and the advice you get from your counselor to overcome these barriers.

Adapted from *Get Clients Now: A 28-Day Marketing Program for Professionals and Consultants* by CJ Hayden. Amacom, $19.95.

your core message

Remember back in Chapter 4 when we had you develop your elevator speech? Now we are going to take that tool to the next level. To review, this is the formula for an elevator speech.

My name is _____. I am a health counselor. I work with _____

(target market) _____

who (what you help your target market with) _____

This is a dynamic way to introduce yourself, but it's only the first level. Quite often, after this introduction, people will want to know more about how you work with your clients. At this time, you can explain that you work with clients in a six-month program designed for their individual needs in which you introduce them to new foods, teach healthy cooking and healthy shopping techniques, and support your clients to maintain healthy, active lifestyles. You should then a question that will make them think about how they could benefit from your services.

Something of great consequence to all your potential clients is what we call WIIFM, which stands for "What's in it for me?" This is the basic question that all potential clients want answered. If you can answer this question for them, they will be interested in becoming a client. To help potential clients understand the benefits of your program, you can ask, "So, for example, what is your main health concern at the moment?" When they respond, you can share with them how you've worked with other clients who had similar concerns by looking at how what they ate affected their health. You can then offer this person a free one-hour consultation with you to discuss their concerns further and see firsthand how you work with your clients.

Do not overlook the importance of explaining how clients benefit from your program. For example, a heath counselor who works with busy professional women who want to eat well and have more energy might mistakenly say, "I offer a six-month program that includes detailed recommendations, a health food store tour, cooking classes, books and handouts." This statement does not tell anyone about how these services actually help the busy professional women. A more effective way to present this information would be to say, "I work with busy professional women to incorporate healthier, more home-cooked foods into their lives. All my clients experience reduced stress and increased energy."

Your core message includes your elevator speech along with a specific description of the many benefits your clients gain from working with you. You will find that you adapt your message slightly, according to whom you are speaking with. For example, if the person who is asking you about your business is overweight, you might add that your clients also lose weight.

A significant disadvantage you face is dealing with the lack of knowledge on the part of the general public about the importance of health. Many people don't realize how much better they will feel if they start eating healthier foods and adopting different, more health-promoting lifestyle choices. Your marketing efforts should involve educating people around the importance of what you do. Don't assume that anyone knows what you do as a health counselor. Explain to people how you work with clients and how those clients will benefit from your services for the rest of their lives! You can do this in your articles and brochure, on your website, at your workshops and at networking events.

filling the pipeline

Marketing is a numbers game. You often have to meet, contact and connect with many people to generate an actual client. For example, you might need to meet the receptionist at a spa, then the manager, then the events coordinator when booking a workshop. At the workshop you meet all the attendees. One of the attendees may refer a friend to you who becomes a client. That is the fifth person who you've interacted with before signing this particular client. Other times, you may run into a stranger at a health food store who becomes a client right away. Anyone you meet could become a client, refer a great client to you, or know of a location or business where you could lead a workshop. The truth is you never know where your next client may come from, but the more people who know you are a health counselor, the more quickly your client base will grow. "Filling the pipeline" means finding ways to meet and connect with new people.

The concept of filling the pipeline comes from *Get Clients Now!* by CJ Hayden. In this book, she outlines her marketing and sales system for getting clients. The first step is to fill the pipeline. According to her principles you should focus on this stage of marketing if you are brand new in business, do not have enough people to call, have called all your prospects in the past 30 days or your prospects don't need or can't afford you. At this point you need to increase visibility and outreach. Some ways to do this are to lead a workshop, attend an event or write an article for the local paper. If you want to have a booming business as a health counselor, your goal should be to have a constant stream of initial Health Histories. To produce this desired outcome, you will need to consistently add people to your pipeline.

Guidelines for filling your pipeline:
- Always follow up with potential clients.
- Research places near you where potential clients hang out: gyms, spas, schools, religious centers, bookstores, etc.
- Lead workshops at least once a month in various places so you are always in front of a new audience: schools, your church or temple, community centers, corporations, etc. Think big!
- Find subtle ways to incorporate your work as a health counselor into conversations with friends and acquaintances.
- Continue gathering phone numbers to call.
- Master outreach: newsletters, phone calls and emails to potential clients and/or referral partners.
- Increase visibility: get published, lead more workshops and add people to your newsletter recipient list.
- Try to create an association with a pre existing company, school, doctor's office, hospital or organization that will give you consistent access to all the new people who walk through their doors.

Once you have mastered filling your pipeline for now (knowing that you will always have to put effort into it), follow through with all the people in your pipeline. Add them to your newsletter recipient list, send them emails to check in, invite them to workshops and cooking classes, and keep them updated on your programs and referral systems. It can take many newsletters or multiple meetings before people are ready to work with you or send you referrals. Keep in touch with all of your contacts and stay visible. Eventually, you want everyone in your pipeline to be so impressed by who you are and the work you are doing that they share it with people they know and, consequently, clients seek you out.

referral systems

Clients like to see professionals who come recommended by someone they already know. Not many people pick their doctors, dentists and massage therapists out of a phone book. You know how when you go to a doctor, and you need a test that they can't perform, they tell you a doctor who can? That is a referral system. Almost all health professionals have referral systems, because they are an effective way of getting new clients.

As a health counselor, you can set up referral systems with doctors, chiropractors, acupuncturists, personal trainers, massage therapists and anyone else you can think of who has clients who might be interested in your services. Directly asking for referrals is common practice among healthcare providers, so you need not be shy.

The first step to setting up a referral system is to make an appointment with someone who you think would be a good referral partner. Maybe it's a chiropractor, doctor or yoga instructor. Then, at the end of your appointment, you can mention that you really enjoyed working with them, and ask if it would be okay to send your clients to see them as well. They will probably ask what you do, and you will respond, "I am a health counselor. I work with (target market) who (what you help your target market with). A lot of my clients are looking for a good (chiropractor, doctor, yoga instructor). Here are some of my brochures. If any of your clients are interested in learning more about how their food affects their health, please feel free to have them call me. I'd also be happy to extend a free consultation to you so that you can become familiar with my services. "

If you already have an established relationship with someone who you'd like to invite to become a referral partner, it may be appropriate to ask that person over for tea or a meal and discuss how you might be able to help each other out. Or you can send your press kit in the mail with a personalized letter inviting the person to create a referral system with you. However our experience shows that talking face to face is more effective than sending materials in the mail.

It's important that you genuinely like and trust the people who become your referral partners. You will be sending your clients to them, and you want your clients to have a good experience.

This is how it works. Let's say you've set up a referral system with a chiropractor and a client is looking for one. Give them your partner's phone number. Then call or send a card to the chiropractor letting them know that your client is coming to see them. Or, after the appointment, send a card thanking them for taking good care of your client and telling them that you look forward to future referrals.

If they send you someone first, send them a small thank-you gift in return. Mailing a gift, no matter how small, will make a strong impression. You could give them a book—maybe the Integrative Nutrition book so they can read more about what you do as a health counselor—a gift certificate to amazon.com or a personalized card.

informal referrals

Think of everyone you know. Now think of everyone they know. You have just started this new, incredible business. Today, the public tends to be skeptical. Hearing about a skilled professional first hand makes a big difference in the decision to call someone. We like everyone from our doctor to our accountant, from our house cleaner to our dry cleaner and our massage therapist to our hair dresser to come on a recommendation from someone we know. That's a lot of people. And you want the people you know to tell everyone they know that you have just started this new, incredible business.

There is no better, more cost-effective way of marketing than word of mouth. Your current clients, friends and family can become an effective marketing team for you by telling people they know about your services. To encourage this, you can create a referral structure for nonprofessionals.

Take a moment now and make a list of 20 health professionals in your area who you could partner with. Use the Internet, ask for ideas from everyone you know and check out the phone book.

1. _____

2. _____

3. _____

4. _____

5. _____

6. _____

7. _____

8. _____

9. _____

10. _____

11. _____

12. _____

13 _____

14 _____

15. _____

16 _____

17. _____

18. _____

19. _____

20. _____

Start with the first person on the list and work your way down. Make contact and give them your referral pitch. It may take a few months to hit everyone on this list, so be patient. Certainly, there has to be at least one person on this list who will be thrilled to create a referral system with you.

referral-building tactics

- Attend meetings and seminars: a good way to meet people because they also came to meet people.
- Schedule office visits: make a date to visit your potential referral partner.
- Serve on committees: this is a relationship-building strategy as well as a visibility strategy.
- Volunteer or trade services: offer free Health Histories to all referral partners (perhaps you'd like to barter your six-month program with some of them).
- Share resources: you can share an office space with massage therapists or other health professionals, or share your contacts and email lists with them.
- Collaborate on projects: you can put together a wellness event with people who you'd like to add to your referral network.

Adapted from *Get Clients Now: A 28-Day Marketing Program for Professionals and Consultants* by CJ Hayden. Amacom, $19.95.

Talk to the social butterfly in your group of friends, your hairdresser, a local real estate agent, a restaurant owner and other people who are well connected. All of these people should know what you do so they can spread the word in their circles. The best way to fill them in is to invite them to a complimentary Health History. At the end of the Health History, they may sign up and they may not. If they do, great! Inevitably, they will start to change and people around them will want to know why. If they don't sign up, that's okay too. You can tell them that you are taking on new clients, and if they know of anyone who might be interested in working with you, they should send them to you. At this time, you can tell them about your referral policy.

Even if you aren't comfortable with pitching your services to your close friends and family, you can invite them for a Health History, letting them know you want the practice. Once the Health History is complete, you don't need to try to close the deal. Simply ask them how it was for them. Let them know that you really appreciate their time and that you enjoyed your meeting. You can casually mention that you are looking for clients, and that if they know anyone who might be interested in hiring you, they can send them your way and you will take great care of them.

Your referral policy might involve giving the same gift to everyone who refers clients to you, or you can do it on a case-by-case basis. For instance, you might give them $50, a book or a gift certificate to amazon.com for every person they refer to you who signs up for your six-month program. Or, if they refer two clients, you offer them a massage. If it's a close friend or family member, it might be appropriate for you to treat them to lunch or dinner. Do whatever feels right to you. Everyone likes to be appreciated, and by your giving gifts when people refer clients to you, you can be certain that they will remember you and most likely continue to send clients your way.

public relations

One of the most effective ways to spread the word about your business is by getting attention from the press. Press attention gives instant credibility to your business. Many graduates have appeared on radio shows, written newspaper articles, had stories about them in the press and even appeared on television. These are great opportunities to increase your visibility and fill your pipeline.

Getting PR may take a little bit of research. Do some investigation into your local press. What television shows feature stories about health? Is there a popular magazine that lists the events going on in your town for the week or the month? What are all the different print publications that your target market might read? What is a hot topic in the news right now, and how can you relate it to your business? Health and wellness are huge issues in the press—everything from obesity to prescription drugs, from Medicare to the latest nutritional supplement is explored.

Contact the media to let them know you are an expert in the field of health and nutrition, and that you'd like to share your knowledge. If possible, find a contact person within the organization and ask them for the protocol to submit a story or get interviewed. Some people will prefer to speak with you first, while others won't speak with you until they have seen your press kit or other information. Snail mail, telephone, email, fax and personal delivery are all functional resources when approaching the media. If you send them a press release or a press kit, it's always best to let them know that you are sending them something, so they are looking out for it when it arrives.

After getting any kind of PR, send a thank-you letter and maybe a small gift to your contact person at the organization. Let them know that you truly appreciate them and that you would love to work together again in the future.

Ways to get free PR:
- Create a health fair in your town and let the press know about it.
- Organize a charity event for a local hospital.
- Offer to write an article for a local newspaper.
- Volunteer your expertise for a radio show.
- Give a workshop at a local school.
- Post articles on the web, always including a link to your website.
- Create a blog.
- Contact organizations that you are a member of and offer to write an article. (Your high school, college, religious or spiritual group is probably looking for members who are up to something.)
- Get involved with a political issue such as school food or government restrictions on supplements.
- Have the places where you do workshops send your materials to their clients and customers.
- Contact your local television station and let them know what you are doing and that you'd be happy to share your expertise with their viewers.
- Lead workshops. Speaking in front of an audience makes you an expert.

writing press releases

A press release is a one-page announcement prepared for distribution to the media about you, your services and, if applicable, a particular event. You want to give journalists information that is useful, clear, to the point and interesting.

Here are steps you can follow to write a press release for a workshop:

- On your computer, design a one-page listing. At the top of the page, use the heading "For Immediate Release" or "Press Release." Below this, place your name and your contact number.
- Design a catchy title such as "Eating Sugar the Right Way" or "Increasing Your Energy Forever." Your title should grab attention and be persuasive. The more unique, the more interest people will show. Place this in bold and center it on the page. You can use all caps as a way to make it further stand out.
- Write the date of the release and the city of origin (e.g., April 16, 2007—New York, NY) .
- In the body of the release, the first paragraph contains, in brief detail, what the press release is about.
- The second paragraph describes what makes your workshop unique and interesting. Don't "sell," just make it stand out by educating readers about the event. Use stimulating text and intriguing details.
- Provide the actual event details in the second paragraph as well, such as the date, location and time.
- The third paragraph should be a one- or two-sentence summary about you, the workshop presenter.
- Include your contact information at the end.
- The content of the press release, beginning with the date and city of origin, should be typed in a clear, basic font and be double-spaced.

Make it fun, timely and accurate. Throw in a fact or two to add credibility. In addition to announcing workshops, you can also design press releases about you, your work in your community or your health counseling practice.

After you send the release, follow up! Call your contacts, confirm that they received the release, and answer any questions they have. Tell them you are interested in having this release considered for publication or announcement, and ask what the steps are to make that happen. Be courteous and professional. They may or may not publicize you or your event, but at least you are developing relationships with key individuals in the media. Relationship building is essential in promoting your business. Keep these people on your contact list, and continue to send them information.

press kits

A press kit, sometimes called a media kit, is simply an information packet about a service or person. It is kind of like an extensive resume that describes your services as a health counselor, provides a biography of you, shares testimonials or references, and allows potential clients or partners to have an overview of your work. The goal is to grab the reader's attention and make a lasting impression.

Who to distribute press kits to:
- the media
- referral partners
- doctors' offices or other complementary practitioners
- spas or other locations where you'd like to be affiliated
- organizations where you want to lecture or do workshops
- key people in the community—those that have access to others
- corporations where you'd like to do a workshop or set up a group program

Composing your Press Kit:
- Use a high-quality folder with pockets on each side and a space for holding your business card. Include your bio and brochure, as well as any flyers for upcoming workshops.
- Include a cover letter addressed to your contact person. It is best to have a pre existing relationship with someone or have a referral since this will speed up the process and heighten your chances of success. In the letter, remind them of the reason for your sending the kit, describe what you have included in the packet, and add a few nice comments about how you are excited about the prospect of working with them. Provide your contact information and tell them you will follow up with them in the following week.
- Include one to two pages that describe health counseling. You can use the text from the website provided to you by the school. Write about your approach to health and wellness, the various workshops you offer and the benefits of this work to your clients. Be creative, be concise and use bullet points to make important information stand out. Customize all information to the person or organization you are addressing. If you are writing to a corporation, for example, include information about your corporate workshops and talk about the benefits to companies who provide wellness education at work, like reduced absenteeism, reduction in health care benefit costs and healthier, happier employees.
- You can also include a sample newsletter or an interesting, relevant article that you or someone else has written.
- It can be helpful to add testimonials and references from current or past clients or other people who have great things to say about you and your work.

Once you have sent your press kit, you must follow up. Contact the person, confirm that they received the packet, and ask if they have any questions about the material. During this call, you should request an in-person meeting to discuss what opportunities exist for you to share your knowledge and expertise with their organization. Use this as an opportunity to build relationships.

bio example

Jane Smith is a Certified Health Counselor and loving mother of two. She decided to become a Health Counselor to fulfill her passion of working with children and parents to improve their health and build vibrant families.

Jane received her training at the Institute for Integrative Nutrition in NYC and is certified by the AADP. She offers individual health and nutrition counseling to parents and families, is a group workshop presenter and a published author.

your bio

When you do workshops or present yourself to a corporation, doctor's office, wellness center or exercise studio, you will often be asked about your background and qualifications. This is the purpose of your bio. It is a portal into your life experience and a condensed version of your career history. It provides your readers with insight into who you are. It can demonstrate your credibility and detail what sets you apart from others.

You should include the bio on all your marketing materials, including brochures, newsletters and flyers.

In most cases, your bio will only be a few sentences. After all, your marketing materials should be more about your clients than about you. The bio should be short, relevant and to the point. It is helpful to have a friend or colleague edit and proofread your bio for readability and grammar.

Your bio may include:
- your education
- awards you have gotten
- something personal about you
- special associations you may belong to
- your mission statement or business philosophy
- any specialized training, certification or licensing
- experience you've had (mostly relevant to what you're doing today)

Use the space below to brainstorm for your bio. Don't worry about complete sentences or perfect grammar. Just get the ideas flowing!

Where were you born and raised?

What is your education, special training, certification, licensing (HC and AADP)?

_____

_____

_____

What associations do you belong to?

_____

_____

_____

What awards have you received?

_____

_____

_____

What unusual experiences have influenced you?

_____

_____

_____

What sets you apart from everyone else? What's something fun, unique, interesting or quirky about you?

_____

_____

_____

What specifically do you provide for your clients?

_____

_____

advertising

You are probably wondering what the difference is between marketing and advertising. The answer lies in money. If you pay to spread the word about your business—either on the Internet, in a magazine or on the radio—that is advertising. If you write an article for a magazine or get interviewed on the radio without paying anyone, that is marketing. Two-thirds of the small businesses in America today operate without any advertising, using marketing alone.

Although some of our graduates find that advertising brings them a few clients each month, we have found that it is not generally effective for health counselors. People are more likely to work with someone they have met or been referred to, and consumers are so overwhelmed with ads that they often don't remember them.

If you do advertise, your best bet is to take out a small ad in a local trade journal or in a healthy living publication. Taking out a classified ad is an easy and inexpensive way to try it out.

internet promotion

Almost every business, from the corner bakery to major corporations, is harnessing the power of the Internet to market themselves. It is important to stay current with your marketing strategies as a health counselor, and find simple yet effective ways to use the Internet to your advantage.

Begin by using the website we give you. Make sure you put the URL on your business card, and list it in every letter and email you send. You can also send your URL to all of your contacts and referral partners, letting them know you have a site with valuable information about your services. Your website can educate potential clients, provide them with additional information after an in-person meeting, and motivate them to take action to find out more about you.

Talk about your website when you give workshops since having one shows you to be credible and organized. Mention it in your newsletter. You can promote your services and have readers visit your site for more detailed information and to learn how to schedule a Health History. Additionally, you can ask your colleagues and referral partners to mention your work and your website address in their newsletters and on their websites.

At some point, you may also choose to develop your own website. Use a qualified and trained web designer, as your site should be professional and persuasive. We caution you again not to spend all your time and money designing a fancy website, however. Marketing is important, but getting out there doing this work and meeting people is more important.

Try this experiment, if you haven't already: google yourself and see what comes up on the net. If nothing comes up, or if the first few hits are not related to health counseling, you may want to increase your visibility on the web. People today google everything. If you meet a prospective client and tell them all about your business, and then they can't find any information about you on the web, they may question your credibility. Increasing your visibility on the web is easy. You can write an article for a website and be sure to include your full name, website and contact information. You can also hire a newsletter company to send out your newsletter each month and archive your past newsletters on the web for you. Webvalence, the company we recommend for newsletter services, will do this at no charge.

Another way to promote yourself online is to join online networks such as friendster and myspace. Cleverly write about your new career as a health counselor using these services. You can also reconnect with old friends and acquaintances. If they are interested, you can invite them for a Health History.

Consider creating a blog, which is short for web log. A blog is a kind of online journal in which you can write about yourself and whatever else you wish. If you are going to use this as a marketing tool, update your blog regularly to provide current health-related information. That way, if someone is searching for that information on the web, they will come to your blog and learn about what you do. This is probably the fastest way to get you up on the web. Go to www.blogger.com or www.typepad.com to learn more about how to create your own blog. It's quite simple. You'll just need a photo, your bio and the ability to regularly update your blog.

If you are computer savvy and want to maximize the benefits of Internet advertising, you can certainly do that. You can purchase banners on other people's websites that display a catch phrase and your contact information. You can buy certain words from search engine companies so that your website comes up on the right-hand side of the page when people search for those particular words. So, for example, if you purchased the words "holistic" and "nutrition," your website would come up when someone typed those words into the search engine. Your choice of key words to purchase is crucial, and you'll have to pay the search engine company each time someone clicks on your link. (The links that come up on the right are paid for. The ones that come up on the left are not paid for, but are generated from the search engine algorithm that factors in the content on your site and its domain name.) You can create great content on your site so that search engines pick it up and other sites want to provide a link to your website. Open Directory will list you on multiple search engines. Please visit http://www.dmoz.org/add.html and follow their instructions. Microsoft has a fee-based service (approximately $49 per year) available to list your site on several search engines, and to manage how effective your site is on the web. Visit www.bcentral.com for more information.

Having your URL appear in website listings is a complicated process, and it entails having the proper key words and code (programming behind your web pages) embedded in the text of your site. Again we recommend that you work with an experienced professional who can design the pages for you and optimize them so that you get maximum exposure.

To learn more about increasing traffic to your website, there are many books you can read or you can simply type "increase website traffic" into a search engine and see what comes up.

What are some ways that you want to enhance your business presence on the Web?

_____

_____

_____

_____

references

You will find that some potential clients—individuals, corporations and organizations—want to hear from people who are familiar with your work. They are interested in working with you, but want to get a second or third opinion before hiring you as their health counselor or workshop presenter. This is when it is useful to have references on file.

After working with clients and organizations—especially those who were raving fans—ask them to write a two- to four-sentence paragraph highlighting your unique qualities and the benefits they received as a result of your work together. Build lasting relationships with these people and organizations because they will become your professional references. Maintain communication, send them your newsletter, keep them up to date on what is happening with your business, and invite them to some of your workshops and seminars. This way if they are asked about you, they have had recent communication and know the latest news about your business.

If you lack experience in a certain area that you'd like to break into—such as corporate workshops or leading school seminars—donate your services for the first few times. Gain experience, build relationships and collect references. You can add all these references to your bio and press kit.

Create a reference handout that includes client feedback, a list of organizations where you have presented workshops, and any other education or achievement that is relevant. Perfect references are past clients or clients currently in your six-month program, referral partners, organizations where you've led workshops and corporate clients. If you do not have many references at this time, think back to your education, work experience and achievements. What people could vouch for your skills as a health counselor? Perhaps an old friend or a family member who is familiar with how much you know about food or a fellow student from Integrative Nutrition could write your first references. Ideally, your references are people who have direct experience with you as a health counselor, but that will come with time. You do not need to put the contact information for your references on your handout if you do not feel ready to do so; simply note that they are available upon request.

List some people or organizations that could be your references:

1. _____

2. _____

3. _____

4. _____

5. _____

6. _____

client testimonials

When your current and past clients share their success stories, potential clients relate to you and your work. Hearing about the success that other people have had in your six-month program will motivate potential clients to want to work with you.

how to gather and use testimonials:

- Think about your best clients, those who have had the greatest success and achieved tangible results. They may be current or past clients.
- Contact these clients, tell them how much you enjoyed working with them and let them know that you are looking for some testimonials.
- If they agree to do it, thank them and let them know what your deadline is. It is best to give people about a week.
- Have them write one to two paragraphs about working with you, the results they achieved, where they were before they met you and where they are now.
- Edit their text and check grammar and spelling.
- Show the client for their approval.
- Place the testimonial on one page, with the client's name, age and profession at the top. Use a picture of them if they are comfortable. If they are worried about confidentiality, just use their first name.
- Upload your testimonials to your website.
- Gather as many testimonials as you can and store them electronically.
- Create a binder full of all your testimonials to show potential clients, organizations and referral partners.
- Arrange several testimonials on one page to hand out to workshop attendees as a quick reference.
- Have organizations you worked for or where you held workshops write testimonials for you.
- Include a testimonial or two on all of your marketing materials, newsletters, brochures, flyers and press kits.

Who are some people you know of who could write you a testimonial?

1. _____

2. _____

3. _____

4. _____

5. _____

6. _____

7. _____

writing

Writing articles, newsletters and columns is a great tool to gain visibility and generate publicity about your practice. Being a published author demonstrates that you have knowledge, while assigning authority to your name and your business. It allows you to communicate with many potential clients and spread your message to hundreds, if not thousands, of people. Writing an article or column in a specific periodical is an excellent way to reach your target market, publicize your business and position yourself as an expert.

Start practicing writing in your own monthly newsletter. Notice what topics you most enjoy writing about and what content comes the easiest to you. Perhaps you love writing recipes or you prefer to write about primary food. Write about what you know best. You can write about anything really. Once you have some writing experience under your belt, you can start to send articles to local newspapers, magazines and Internet ezines. Perhaps you'd even like to write a monthly or weekly health advice column.

Don't rule out writing as a marketing method simply because you don't think you are a good writer. There are many writing coaches and copy editors out there who would be happy to help you for as little as $15 an hour.

When approaching publications, you can either send them an article and see if they'd like to publish it, or make contact with them and say that you'd like to write an article for their readers. Suggest a topic you think is pertinent and see how they respond. Once a topic is agreed upon, find out your deadline and hit the keyboard.

Tips for writing effective articles:
- Write about topics that will interest your target audience and relate to their needs.
- Write about topics that you know personally.
- Don't give away too much in the article. Give people just enough so they feel they learned something, but they want to know even more.
- Make the article easy to read, with useful content.
- Spell check, edit and proofread. It's usually best to have someone else proofread for you.
- If possible, become a regular writer for one or more publications so that over time you build relationships with your readers.
- Do research to find out what the hot topics are for your target audience.
- Practice makes perfect. The more you practice writing, the easier it gets.

How to write an article:
- Identify a problem your target audience is experiencing.
- Consider how you can offer a solution to their problem.
- Brainstorm ideas for the article on a pad of paper or your computer, writing down everything that comes to mind.
- Create an outline, a master layout of your article from start to finish that contains your thesis, supporting ideas and information, and closing paragraph concept.
- Think of a catchy title to grab readers' attention.

- In the first paragraph, ask a question or two that helps the readers relate to your article and has them interested in reading further (e.g., "Are you tired of being addicted to sugar?", "Do you have a huge decrease in energy every afternoon?").
- Include interesting information, valuable facts and some pieces of simple advice in the body of the article.
- Use humor if possible or keep the tone light, as many people take health too seriously and are looking for a new approach.
- End the article with a conclusion, as well as an invitation to call you or visit your website to schedule a free Health History.

Edit the article two to three times or more before publishing, making sure you have enough time in between edits to come to the page with a fresh, sharp mind.

How to distribute your article:
- Send it to your contact list.
- Place it on your website or in your newsletter.
- Build a database of editors. Identify magazines, newspapers, online publications and other periodicals that relate to your expertise and target market. Call those publications on your list, get the email addresses and contact information of editors who are responsible for the area you write about (health, nutrition, healing), and find out who is in charge of article submissions.
- Send a cover letter, along with a copy of your article, to those contacts. Give them a week or so to review, then follow up with a phone call to talk, answer questions and see what possibilities exist for being published in their periodical.
- Send extra articles to your colleagues and referral partners. Have them distribute the article, along with your contact information, to their mailing list.

writing and publishing a book

Starting a new career as a health counselor—whether it is full time or part time—is a huge undertaking. If you are committed to growing your health counseling business, maintaining focus is crucial. If writing a book is something you desire to achieve, we definitely support you in this endeavor. However we recommend that you wait to write a book until after you have a few years of health counseling experience. Writing a book is an enormous project. It will demand a lot of your time and energy. Your experience of working with clients will be instrumental in guiding you towards what kind of book you'd like to produce and the most effective way to introduce your material to the public.

Being an author of a published book is a major accomplishment and one that, although not easy, is incredibly rewarding. Writing a book is a great way to increase your credibility, boost self-esteem and get respect. Anyone who doubted your ability to be successful as a health counselor will eat their words when you give them your first book.

Although we do not recommend you write a book at this time, you can begin to think about what you might like to write about. Think of a subject that you are an expert in and that people want to know about. These days, narrow topics are the best. People want specified information. Writing a book about nutrition is very broad. What are your specialties? Who is your target market? What information would be most useful to them?

Once you know what you'd like your book to be about, create a detailed outline. This outline should contain all the major topics in your book, along with the supporting information you need to get your point across most effectively. You can organize your outline by chapter or by topic. Know that your outline will change once you start to write.

When your outline is in good shape, you can start to investigate publishing. Your two main options are to self-publish your book or to find a publishing house. There are benefits and drawbacks to each, of course. In self-publishing, you maintain all the control of your book—the content, design and marketing scheme. The major drawback is that you foot the bill. Another thing to keep in mind is that you will have to do all your own marketing and sales. But you also get to keep all of the profit. When going with a publisher, they pay for everything and invest their resources into marketing your book. However, the publisher also has final say over the content, look and feel of your book. There are certain ideas they may not let you print. You will only receive a portion of the profits when your book is sold through a publishing house.

If you decide to self-publish, you can start to write your manuscript. When your book is about half done, you should find a book designer and printer you would like to use. You will also have to secure a proofreader and indexer. There are also self-publishing services, such as www.authorhouse.com, that provide editing, design, promotion, printing and marketing services for a fee. Check bookstores and the Internet for many reference guides on how to self-publish.

If you'd like to work with a publishing house, you should write your book proposal shortly after completing your outline. You do not want to write your book first because the publisher may steer you in a different direction than you would go on your own. Know that there are many books out there about how to write a killer book proposal.

Brainstorm possible topics for your first book:

1. _____

2. _____

3. _____

4. _____

5. _____

branding

Quick, think of Coca-Cola. Now think of Nike. Now Verizon. All of these companies have a clear and consistent brand. You know what they look like, you know what they offer and you can recognize their logos anywhere. Some people mistakenly believe that they key to branding is putting a lot of resources into advertising. Actually, the best way to build a solid, recognizable brand is to build a look and feel to your business and consistently deliver high-quality services.

Branding is not a necessary element of having a successful health counseling business. Many graduates do not even have a logo or brochure for their practices and their practices are full. If developing a brand is overwhelming or uninteresting to you at this time, skip it. You can always come back to this section in the future.

If you are interested in building a recognizable brand, start with your company name. Then create an attractive logo that complements your company name and uses colors that inspire you. Ask yourself if your materials send a clear, consistent message about who you are and the services you offer.

Start to use your logo and company name on all your materials, from your business cards to your newsletter, from the handouts given at lectures to your website. You want to increase familiarity. The more people see your brand, the more they will begin to accept your business's credibility.

finding time for marketing

Sometimes people say they don't have time to do marketing. What they usually mean is that they feel blocked or confused about how to do marketing in an effective way. Marketing is so important. It helps people find you, so that you can help them. Here are some tips for how to make time for marketing:

- Make a list of your marketing tasks and identify what you need to do to reach your goals.
- Commit to marketing tasks and then schedule them. For example, if you send out a newsletter, choose a day in your calendar each month to create it and send it out. Then stick to it.
- Pick times for marketing and do your marketing activities at the same time and day each week. Make it your marketing hour or marketing day. For example, Monday afternoons could be your time to call wellness centers and corporations about doing talks and to send out your press kits.
- Do one thing at a time. Rome was not built in day. Taking on too much at once could thwart your efforts. Focus on one area of marketing at a time: either writing, networking, teaching workshops or boosting your presence on the Internet. Chunk each task down into smaller tasks. Once one task is complete, you can add something new.
- Give to others. Give of your time, materials and newsletters. When you give, you will receive.
- Build a group of people to support you with your marketing. You can use your counselor, fellow students and helpful friends and family

developing a marketing plan

To help motivate you to stay on top of your marketing, here we are going to have you develop a basic marketing plan. Think of your marketing plan as a highly organized strategy for your marketing procedures. The purpose of this plan is to choose the methods that will best support your business goals, while staying within your budget. A professional marketing plan usually includes analysis of your target market, how you'd like to be positioned in the market, an analysis of your competition, past attempts at marketing and their success rates, and your current strategy and expenses.

Marketing requires adaptation and innovation. One month your newsletter could bring in a few initial consultations. The next month you might want to design and send out a holiday postcard to everyone in your pipeline, letting them know your New Year's discounts. Consider your marketing plan as a work in progress.

How many clients do you have now?

_____

How many clients do you want to have by graduation?

_____

Who is your target market?

_____

_____

How would you like to be positioned in the market?

_____

_____

Who are your competitors?

_____

_____

_____

_____

_____

_____

Describe your past marketing efforts, how effective they were and how much money and time you put into them.

_____

_____

_____

_____

_____

Make a list of marketing techniques you would like to try, such as getting on the radio, publishing an article, increasing word of mouth and referrals, attending health fairs, boosting your online presence or any other concept from this chapter and Chapter 4.

_____

_____

_____

_____

_____

How and when do you plan to implement these techniques?

_____

_____

_____

_____

_____

What day of the week would you like to designate as your marketing day?

_____

What hours on this day will you spend on your marketing materials and events?

_____

six marketing tips

You Can Avoid Advertising

More than two-thirds of the profitable small businesses in the U.S. operate without advertising. Concentrate on creating a high-quality product that your customers will rave about, spreading the word. Plan marketing events that keep customers involved and get positive media attention for your business.

Drive Customers by Need, Price and Access

Need: When you're considering how to market, determine why customers need your products.
Price: Consumers like prices that are clear, easy to understand and not hidden.
Access: If cost and quality are equal between you and another provider, customers usually patronize the one that's easiest to access. How easy is it for customers to find you?

Go Guerrilla

Guerrilla marketing requires time, energy and imagination, but not a lot of money. Jay Levinson's *Guerilla Marketing* was the first marketing book aimed squarely at small businesses. Levinson is a proponent of simple marketing devices, such as brochures, signs and low-cost public events like seminars and free consultations.

Marketing Is a Sensory Experience

Marketing is a lot like dating. You're trying to get somebody interested and then retain their interest while you figure out if you should work together. Much of the attraction is based on the sensory experience—how your business looks, smells and the sense of order it instills. Don't underestimate the importance of a clean and uncluttered environment.

Yes, the Customer Is (Almost) Always Right

One of the least expensive, most effective marketing techniques is to adopt customer-friendly policies. Your customer service program may include mailing cards, listening without interruption to any complaints, or providing extras for your clients.

Words That Sell

When writing copy for your marketing materials, use words that sell and inspire. Make the most effective use of your words. Look at your copy from the customer's perspective. Don't fill your copy with empty statements or superfluous information. Using too many superlatives, such as "amazing," "incredible" and "fantastic" may hinder your credibility. You may want to check out Richard Bayan's *Words That Sell* for more information on how to write effective marketing copy.

Adapted from *Whoops! I'm in Business: A Crash Course in Business Basics* by Richard Steim and Lisa Guerin. Nolo, $19.99.

month-by-month marketing and seminar ideas

Month:	Concepts to Incorporate into Your Marketing Plan
January	New Year's Resolutions
	Getting back on track health-wise
	Back to basics (water, breakfast)
	Hibernation is not just for bears (self-nurturance)
February	Sugar Blues Talks - Valentine's Day!
	Self-Love: You don't need a significant other to celebrate heart day
	Mardi Gras celebrations: colorful and healthful foods to enjoy to your heart's delight
March	Beating the winter blues
	National nutrition month
	Managing seasonal allergies/hay fever
April	Spring cleaning: cleansing and fasting
	Harvest time for grains
May	Mother's Day
	Celebrating your womanhood
	Live/raw foods
	May Day: celebration of fertility (flower baskets/outdoor gathering)
June	Outdoor activities and exercise
	Weight management
	Prepare your body for summer
	Father's Day: celebrating men
July	Summer eating and keeping cool
	Travel time
	Making healthy choices on the road
	Independence Day: multinational celebration
	(U.S., France, Canada, Philippines, Venezuela, Argentina, Belgium, Peru)
August	De-junk your kitchen
	Harvest
September	Back to school
	Snazzy snacking (brown-bagging it is not just for school kids)
	Noshing for energy, taste and fun
	Stocking up your pantry
	Simplifying shopping
	Spirituality connection: Jewish holidays
	Preparation for seasonal change: fall is a typical fasting and detoxification season
October	Deconstructing cravings
	Fall foods
	True Halloween treats, sans refined sugar tricks
	Transition: changing of the leaves, days become shorter
	Vegetarian awareness month
November	Holiday preparation
	Surviving the holidays
	Self-nurturance
	Slowing down with the season/shorter days
	Flu season: boost your immune system
December	Holiday celebrations: Christmas, Hanukkah, Kwanzaa
	Healthy gift-giving
	Eating for energy

seasons in health counseling

An effective way to plan your marketing strategy is to understand which business activities are most effective at which times of the year. The best months for lectures and signing up clients are January, March, April, May, October and November. Plan for this by offering special holiday gift certificates in November and December. Book a lot of public speaking events for early January through May. Likewise, use the summer months to coordinate events for the fall.

December is usually a slow month for health counselors. People are busy with the holidays and are spending a lot of money. It may be in your best interest to hold off doing Health Histories with people until mid-January, once the chaos of the holidays has worn off and regular life has been restored. You may want to use December to work on updating your marketing materials, press kit and website. This is a great time to book workshops and seminars for the coming year as well as schedule some down time or vacation time for yourself. However, there have been health counselors who sign loads of clients in December. Keep your options open.

In the summer, even though many people go on vacation and become more relaxed, you can still be proactive around building your business. Maintain momentum by utilizing unique summer resources. You can lead workshops at summer camps, teach Mommy-and-me cooking classes, organize a weekend retreat to the beach or the woods, attend health fairs or create a group program that meets outside and helps clients get sexy for the beach. Be creative!

Don't forget that part of being a health counselor is walking your talk. Rest, relaxation, fun and play are vital to creating health. Therefore, it is totally okay, in fact it is mandatory, that you take some time off in the summer. Even if you don't go anywhere, it is healthy to take a break from work for a week or two. You can let your clients know in advance that you are going on vacation, and that their program will pick up again when you get back. Explain that this extends the length of their six-month program. By taking time for yourself, you are demonstrating via example the importance of balance to your clients.

doing what comes naturally

When deciding which strategies are most effective for your business, strongly consider what you enjoy doing and what comes naturally to you. Some marketing techniques will be second nature, while others will feel like pulling teeth. Perhaps you don't enjoy writing, but are an excellent cook and love teaching cooking classes. You can ask around at school and on the OEF for another counselor who would like to help you with your writing in exchange for your helping them learn how to teach a great cooking class. If you absolutely hate leading workshops, the people who attend are going to sense it, so it will not be an effective marketing tool for you. You should discover what kind of marketing you enjoy, and do it often. The more natural and creative your marketing techniques, the more success you will encounter.

Please keep in mind that you are your best advertisement. You are your business's walking billboard. Your health and happiness are instrumental in generating business. Don't waste your precious time doing things that make you unhappy. The more you are focused on doing what you love, the more you are out and about looking like your radiant self, the more people will want to know who you are and learn how they can get some of what you've got.

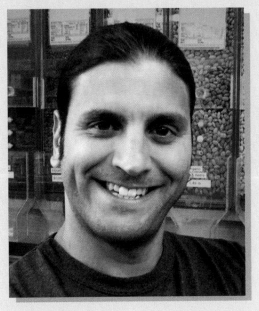

When I decided to come to Integrative Nutrition, I was really struggling. I had no career and was living in an attic apartment with rusty water. I stumbled upon the catalog and felt like I had been guided in some way to find it.

During the school year, I learned about my body, got back into sports, began to cook whole foods and healed my digestive organs. I affiliated with a doctor's office and started seeing clients there. I did free talks at gyms, tanning salons and day spas to promote myself.

I marketed myself using the guidelines the school taught me. It was mostly just getting out there and talking to people. I worked hard in the beginning and it paid off. In the three years since I graduated, I've worked with 150 people in my health counseling program, and I went from that one-bedroom apartment to my own two-story house on the water in Long Island.

Michael Macaluso
Seaford, NY
Michaeljmacaluso@aol.com
2003 Graduate

At the doctor's office I see a lot of diabetics, cardiac patients and senior citizens. I also work with mothers and people with food allergies and sensitivities. By structuring it as a three-month program with weekly sessions, we build a lot of momentum and make changes quickly. We start with the absolute essentials by developing a structured morning routine of deep breathing, stretching, drinking water, movement and eating a healthy breakfast. Once clients have their mornings down, we move on to lunch, snacks and dinner.

I teach my clients to be self-directed, independent thinkers who take control of their own health and rely on their own inner voice, rather than the media. The coolest part about this work is that if I weren't getting paid, I would do it anyway! I am making a big impact in my community because my clients are teaching their kids, friends, families and coworkers about healthy eating.

My best piece of advice is to have your pitch for initial consultations well organized. Make sure you know your program inside and out so you can clearly and concisely explain it to others. Be certain you can communicate what benefits clients can expect from working with you. Speaking with conviction and believing in yourself is what convinces people to work with you, not pieces of paper or letters after your name.

Under no circumstances should you ever quit. Make the commitment now and use the school year to follow through. I didn't have a computer, money or a car when I started. All I had was the education and materials the school gave me, and an unstoppable desire to help people. No matter where you're starting from or what your background is, you can take this education with you anywhere and create a successful practice.

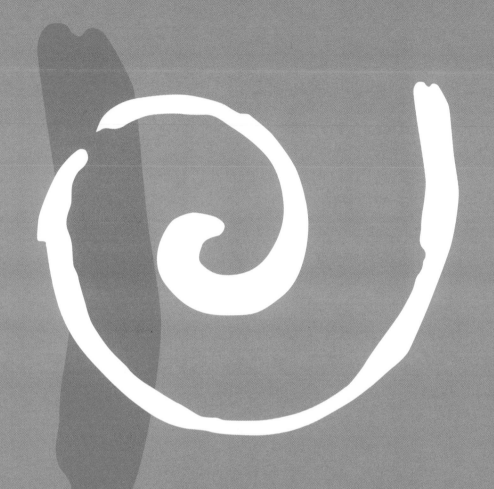

chapter nine

You can't just sit there and wait for people to give you that golden dream; you've got to get out there and make it happen for yourself.

Diana Ross

maintaining momentum

It takes a few years to build a solid business. Don't expect it all to happen overnight. It may seem to you that some of your classmates or our alumni had clients fall into their laps, that they never doubted themselves. This is not the case. Everyone has times when they doubt their ability to do this work. It is the nature of being in business for yourself. What's important is that you push yourself through those times and continue moving forward. Self-motivation—being inspired by what you do and having goals in sight—is necessary for keeping up the work. Keep reminding yourself why you wanted to be a health counselor in the first place. Take constant inventory of the positive influences you are having on your clients, your family and your friends. You are a source of inspiration for your community, and you have so much to offer!

starting where you are

No matter the current shape of your business—if you have zero or 30 clients—accept where you are and move from there. You do not want to be ahead of yourself or behind yourself in any way. For example, if you haven't signed any clients yet, you don't want to focus on building a website or writing a book. Instead, focus your effort on getting Health Histories. Likewise, if you already have a full practice and can't handle any more clients, you don't need to spend hours booking a workshop; your energy is probably better spent on time management and deepening your counseling skills.

Here are some recommended action steps to take, depending on where you are in your business.

if you have no clients:
This is a great place to be because your business can only get better from here. You are at the beginning of creating a career you love, and you have so much to look forward to. Your task now is to fill your pipeline with potential clients by networking in person. Tell people you are a health counselor. Network at business groups and parties. Give talks. Invite people to Health Histories and do as many as you can. The more Health Histories you do, the sooner you will have paying clients.

if you are counseling part time

Continue to focus on marketing yourself in person. Stay visible and in demand so that there is always someone about to sign up with you. This way, when a client finishes a program, you can enroll a new client to fill that slot right away. Give talks, network and make special offers to clients who refer people who sign up with you.

Evaluate how many clients are ideal for you. Are you happy counseling part time? Do you want to eventually go full time? If so, when? Some people are happy counseling only five clients at a time. Others want to counsel ten, 20 or 30 clients. Some new counselors think that if their number of clients plateaus along the way they can't do this work full time. This isn't true. If you want to grow your business, you can. Decide for yourself how many clients are ideal, then increase or decrease your marketing hours, or change your action steps to get the number of clients you want.

if you are counseling full time

At this point you have completed a lot of the basic marketing work it takes to attract clients. You are probably managing a lot of paperwork, people and opportunities. The time you spend on marketing should be limited and focused. Do one powerful marketing activity each day. Or set aside one day a week for marketing and do seven activities.

Put energy into building a sustainable business structure. Manage your time well and increase your level of self-care so you don't burn out. Hire an assistant at $10 to $15 an hour to help you with administrative details. Enlist PR or media relations help so you can get your business out there without having to do all the footwork yourself.

You can also take advantage of passive marketing techniques, where other people find clients for you. Build referral networks with other practitioners so they send potential clients your way. Underpromise and overdeliver for all your clients, so that they become raving fans and spread the word about how fabulous you are.

In Chapter 1 we asked you to set goals for what you want your health counseling business to look like. Have you achieved them?

If so, what led to your success? _____

_____

How do you feel? _____

_____

If not, that's okay too. Take an honest look at why not.

What one obstacle are you committed to overcoming? _____

_____

_____

Have your goals changed, and if so, how? _____

_____

What can you do differently in the future to meet your goals? _____

_____

having fun

If you want your career as a health counselor to be satisfying, you simply must find a way to incorporate having fun into your business. Being an overly serious workaholic who is adamantly attached to changing the world will get old soon enough. Take a step back, enjoy your precious life and find a way to create balance between work and play.

Notice what parts of health counseling bring you the most energy and excitement. Do you absolutely love giving talks? Sending out your newsletter? Leading health food store tours? Whatever you enjoy most, do more of it. Similarly, notice what parts of health counseling drain your energy and do less of those!

What are three parts of health counseling drain your energy?

1. _____

2. _____

3. _____

What are three parts of health counseling that turn you on?

1. _____

2. _____

3. _____

How can you do less of things that drain your energy and more of what you truly enjoy?

1. _____

2. _____

3. _____

ideas for incorporating fun into your practice

- Create arts and crafts projects to do in your client sessions or in your seminars, such as collages, finger painting, candle making, painting pottery or making your own holiday cards.
- Instead of a monthly seminar, take clients out dancing, to karaoke or for a picnic.
- Hold client sessions outside somewhere beautiful.
- Invite exciting guest speakers to your monthly seminars, such as belly dancers, palm readers, fashion experts, feng shui practitioners or creative writing teachers.
- Offer to help your clients de-clutter their home or kitchen. Hold a session at their place and give them tips on how to clean up clutter.
- Make it a goal to laugh at least once in each session. If this is difficult for you, find something that makes you laugh and keep it in your office at all times.

support people

A happy and energized health counselor is one who is getting support—and lots of it. The only way to get the support you need is to ask for it. You can't do everything alone, and by asking for assistance, in both your business and your personal life, your chances of success skyrocket.

Health counseling is a giving profession, meaning you are constantly giving to your clients, prospective clients and probably the majority of the people in your life. To ensure that there is a balance of give and take, you need to create a support structure or system that works for you, a way to recharge your battery and discharge stress. An ideal support structure is made up of everyone in your life. This is a fact: you can never have too much encouragement. And know that it is possible to have everyone – your family, friends, significant other, coworkers and boss—be supportive of who you are and what you are doing. It is a sign of strength to allow others to hold you up, to be vulnerable at times and to take into account the ideas of others.

Who are the five people in your life that support you the most?

1. _____

ways this person supports you:

_____

_____

2. _____

ways this person supports you:

_____

_____

3. _____

ways this person supports you:

_____

_____

4. _____

ways this person supports you:

_____

_____

5. _____

ways this person supports you:

_____

_____

Find a way to appreciate these five people for all they do. Tell them how grateful you are for having them in your life. Explain what they do that you find specifically helpful, and encourage them to keep on doing it! Find ways to make these people more central in your life. And, make sure it is a mutually supportive relationship, where both people benefit.

Now, ask yourself how you might be able to get this kind of support from others. Are there people in your life who you would like to be closer with, but whom you find unsupportive? How can you ask them for the kind of support you need? Or is it time to reduce their role in your life or cut them out? If it is family members who are unsupportive, it is usually best to do whatever is in your power to be on good terms with them, without compromising yourself.

Who are five people who are unsupportive of you or of a certain aspect of the way you live?

1. _____

ways this person is unsupportive:

_____

_____

2. _____

ways this person is unsupportive:

_____

_____

3. _____

ways this person is unsupportive:

_____

_____

4. _____

ways this person is unsupportive:

_____

_____

5. _____

ways this person is unsupportive:

_____

_____

Without a doubt, you are going to come across some people who are unsupportive of your decisions. These people may truly care about you and only want the best for you. If that is the case, communicate with them openly about why you are making the choices you are, and why you really need their support right now. Hear out their concerns, and reply honestly.

It is possible that these unsupportive people may not be the best people for you to have in your life anymore. There are those in this world who are very jealous, who don't want to see their friends doing well. There are also those who are scared of change and prefer everything to stay the same, always. If you are changing—beginning a new career, eating new foods and making different lifestyle choices—you will be challenging their reality. Ask yourself if there are some people who you know in your heart you would be better off without. It is okay to let them go. You are not doing them or yourself any favors by continuing to be a part of a dysfunctional relationship. If breaking off contact seems drastic, you can downgrade your relationship, see them less often and give them less of your energy.

your buddy

The people closest to you may not always be the best support people for your business. As much as they love you, their tolerance for hearing about another Sugar Blues talk or Health History might be low. Your buddy from class is a valuable support person for you because they know where you are coming from, and they are also just starting out as a health counselor. The two of you should meet or speak regularly. Your buddy's duty is to listen to you, celebrate with you, commiserate with you, be your brainstorming partner and keep you focused on achieving your goals. This is also your duty to your buddy.

creating community

An important ingredient to the success of our school is community. As you know by now, many of our students make some of the best friends of their lives while they are here. This happens naturally because the school attracts people who are healthy, happy and who want to do something that inspires them and helps others. We strongly encourage you to take advantage of the community you have here at the school. Meet new people at each class weekend, have lunch with other students, get together outside of class and build relationships. Having other health counselors in your life is priceless. They know how to listen, give good advice and also can support you in your career.

local study chapters

We at the school created local study chapters because we noticed that students truly enjoyed hanging out, getting to know and supporting one another. We highly encourage you to take advantage of this valuable resource. Attend local study chapters held by people in your area, or on the phone. Even better, hold your own local study chapter. Pick a topic related to business and invite however many people you like. During the local study chapter, share business tips, stories, challenges and laughs!

board of directors

A key to success is getting expert advice from supportive people who have more knowledge and experience than you. Corporations, schools and nonprofit foundations accomplish this by having boards of directors who advise them on their business decisions and goal planning. We recommend you create a board of directors for your health counseling business. Your board will share their knowledge, help you make important decisions, give you support, hold you accountable and help you reach new levels of success.

how to create a board of directors

1. Decide whom to invite. You will need between four and six people on your board. Who are your peers and mentors with valuable insight to share? An accountant, lawyer or business professional? A friend who works in marketing? A successful health counselor? Another experienced person in a healing profession?

2. Invite each person them to participate in your business as an advisor. Share with them how committed you are to your business success and how much you value their wisdom and support.

3. Let each person know up front what their time commitment will be: one conference call each month for 30 to 60 minutes. Ask them what are three possible days and times they could meet every month (e.g., every third Tuesday at 5:00 pm). Choose a schedule that works for everyone.

4. Send an email to your entire group, introducing everyone to each other and asking them to mark the meeting schedule on their calendars. It should be the same week, day and time every month.

5. Use www.freeconference.com to schedule the calls. Be sure to send your board the phone number and any necessary access codes.

6. Before each call, choose two or three areas of your business where you need the most support. You could also prepare a summary of your business before each meeting to keep your board up to date on your progress. Make sure you leave time for group brainstorming.

7. Keep meeting regularly. Consistent support is crucial to success. If members need to leave your group, find others to replace them.

8. Appreciate your board. Send thank-you cards and emails or small gifts like amazon.com gift certificates. Let them know how much you value their support.

9. Give back. Offer to be on their boards of directors in return.

Write down the names of five people you want on your board of directors.

1. _____

2. _____

3. _____

4. _____

5. _____

Your board does not have to be arranged in any formal way. The goal is to have regular contact with knowledgeable people who actively support you and your business growth. Set this up however works best for you.

hiring a business coach

If you are clear that you want your business to grow, but you need more guidance on how to make that happen, you might want to hire a business coach. When your sessions end with your health counselor in the spring, your counselor may offer their services to you at a discounted rate. You may choose to take them up on this offer.

A different option would be to hire another health counselor as your coach. We have many graduates who have been practicing successfully for years and offer business coaching to current students and alumni. Most of these people have probably already come and spoken to you during class. Their contact information is on the OEF. They would be delighted to hear from you and tell you about the business coaching that they offer.

mentors

Anyone who has ever had a mentor or been a mentor knows that the mentor-mentee relationship is beautiful. To guide a person through something that you have already experienced, to encourage them, warn them of the roadblocks and tell them they can do it, is an extremely rewarding experience. Likewise, having someone show you the ropes, someone you can confide in and trust, is priceless. Know that there are many people in the Integrative Nutrition community and in the world who would be honored to offer their expertise to you. Your health counselor is one of these people.

Ask yourself if you know someone whose business expertise you admire. Who is someone you aspire to be like? Pick up the phone or turn on your computer, and reach out to this person. Invite them to lunch, let them know that you've just started a new business and you'd love to share some ideas—that you really value their expert opinion.

List here the names of three people who you would like to have as your mentor.

1. _____

2. _____

3. _____

Now devise a plan for making them a part of your life. It might be appropriate to hire this person —if they are a business coach—or maybe you simply work towards building a friendly relationship. Know that you become like the people who you associate with, so surrounding yourself with accomplished, first-rate people is a sure way to invite success.

self-care

A common vice among health counselors is that we can put so much energy into taking care of others we forget or don't have time to take care of ourselves. If you keep up this behavior, you will eventually burn out and have nothing to give anyone. You'll wonder where you went wrong; you may even develop illness.

Your body sends you messages through its ailments, and usually the messages are this: "Take better care of me!" As a health counselor and a human being you must learn to discipline yourself to take care of your mental, physical, emotional and spiritual health.

Take note of the signs your body sends you when you are out of balance, burning the candle at both ends or not taking good enough care of yourself. List the top five ways here:

1. _____

2. _____

3. _____

4. _____

5. _____

Be on alert for these messages. Lovingly listen to them and take the appropriate action to get yourself back into balance.

We encourage you to practice extreme self-care. What do we mean by extreme self-care? At least once a day do something to energize or rejuvenate yourself. This will look different for everyone, and it will look different depending on the day. It may mean getting a massage, going into nature, taking a bubble bath, cooking your favorite meal, going for a walk around the block at work, seeing a movie or whatever pleases you. It may be that you need to do two things a day for yourself, or even three. Hopefully, over time, self-care will become second nature to you, and you won't even consider putting everyone else's needs in front of your own.

stress

Stress has extreme negative effects on our overall health; it causes all sorts of illness, affects sleep and digestion, can lead to depression and lowers the quality of life. Develop reliable and simple ways to reduce stress. Experiment with meditation, hot towel scrubs, drinking more water, herbal tea, running outside or whatever helps you to quiet your mind and feel at peace. Eating well and doing regular physical activity are excellent ways to reduce stress and nurture yourself. Do whatever you need to make these things regular occurences in your life.

What are the main sources of stress in your life at the moment?

1. _____

2. _____

3. _____

4. _____

5. _____

How can you either let go of these causes of stress, or reduce or eliminate the stress they bring into your life? (List two steps for each issue.)

1. _____

_____

2. _____

_____

3. _____

_____

4. _____

_____

5. _____

_____

What are three things you know you can do that help you when you feel stressed?

1. _____

2. _____

3. _____

be your own best manager

- identify your values and operate from them
- clarify your purpose, priorities and goals
- design and implement an effective business plan
- create strategic plans of action
- learn to work smarter—not harder
- eliminate time wasters
- plan your days
- set a schedule and keep it
- take a stretch break every 20 minutes
- be dressed for "work"
- get feedback from colleagues and experts
- collect information: quotes, articles, statistics
- keep your workspace organized
- enhance telephone skills
- follow through with clients
- market your business consistently
- join at least one professional association
- develop powerful networking abilities
- keep accurate records
- be a calculated risk taker
- be willing to move on
- make sure your needs are being met
- exercise regularly
- create a support system
- continue your education
- get out of the house/office EVERY DAY!!!
- take responsibility for yourself
- choose appropriate advisors
- keep things in perspective
- for tasks you hate—delegate (or subcontract)
- respect your mind's and body's cycles
- balance your personal and professional life
- remember, we're all human—we all make mistakes
- acknowledge your accomplishments every day

Excerpted from *Business Mastery: A Guide for Creating a Fulfilling, Thriving Business and Keeping It Successful* by Cherie M. Sohnen-Moe, Sohnen-Moe Associates, Inc, $24.95

time management

Time management is an important skill to have in life, but it is especially critical when you own and operate your own business. Everyone has a different idea of time management. Whatever way you choose to look at it, we all have the same 24 hours in a day. The secret to managing your time effectively is to know how much it is worth and put your time towards the things that are most important to you.

What are your current beliefs about time (not enough of it, goes by too quickly, etc.)?

_____

_____

What were your parents' beliefs and relationships to time?

_____

_____

Where does the majority of your time go?

_____

_____

What are three things you spend time on that aren't important to you?

1. _____

2. _____

3. _____

If you had more time, what would you do with it?

_____

_____

_____

_____

How can you create more time to focus on what is really important to you?

_____

_____

To become strong at time management does not mean that you have to work longer hours; you simply have to work smarter. Most people spend a good portion of their time on things that aren't effective. Working smarter means maximizing your working hours. Use the time you spend working wisely, so that you have more time to enjoy life, relax, have fun, cook, exercise and do whatever else you love.

tips for time management

Know how many hours you want to work each week.

- Identify the times of day when you do your best work.
- Identify the times of day that are difficult for you to work.
- Build your schedule around your personal time cycles: when you work best, when it is best for you to exercise, to eat, to sleep, etc.
- Know your limit—how many hours a day and a week you can work before burning out.
- Acknowledge that there is a time in a day, after working a certain number of hours, when your efforts actually stop being useful.
- Clarify your goals and priorities, and make sure you spend most of your time working towards your biggest goals.
- Identify things you do that do not support your goals, and drop them.
- Make it your job to master the art of being successful in health counseling and staying balanced.

weekly timesheet

When you begin your practice, plan to spend about 75% of your time lining up and doing Health History consultations. The remaining 25% of your time will be spent following up with potential clients, keeping track of them and preparing for your meetings. Once you start signing clients, you'll probably spend about 50% of your time marketing your services and doing Health Histories, 30% of your time meeting with clients, and 20% of your time on follow-up and preparation.

To help you master time management, we've created this weekly timesheet. Keep it, or one like it, in your office or in a journal. Before lunch each day, write in how many hours you spend on each category. Do the same again at the end of your workday. It's a good way to see where you are putting your energy and how long certain tasks take you. You may think that most of your time goes into marketing, but in actuality you may be spending hours upon hours on the Internet. At the end of each week, review this time sheet, making note of where most of your time went. Reflect on it, and decide if this was an effective use of your time. Make the appropriate adjustments in the following week.

weekly timesheet

	Health Histories	Client Sessions	Writing/ Newsletter	Marketing & Networking	Paperwork Phone	Email/ Phone	Other
Monday am							
Monday pm							
Tuesday am							
Tuesday pm							
Wednesday am							
Wednesday pm							
Thursday am							
Thursday pm							
Friday am							
Friday pm							
Saturday							
Sunday							

big rocks

Named after a demonstration performed by a time-management expert, Franklin Covey, Big Rocks is a concept used throughout Integrative Nutrition. In the demonstration, the expert takes a jar and fills it with some big rocks. He asks his students if the jar is full. They say it is. He proceeds to dump gravel into the jar, and shake the jar around so the pieces of gravel fill up the spaces between the big rocks. He asks his students if the jar is full. They respond, "Probably not." Next, he pours sand into the jar, which fills in all the empty spaces between the gravel and the rocks. Again, he asks, "Is the jar full?" The students shout, "No!" Finally, he takes a pitcher of water and pours it into the jar until it is full to the brim. His point is not that you can always fit more into your jar, but that if you don't put in your big rocks first, you'll never get them in at all.

Each Monday morning, everyone on the Integrative Nutrition staff completes their Big Rocks list—an inventory of all the important tasks they are going to accomplish in the coming week, along with how many hours they plan to spend on each one. They list the tasks that take the most amount of time at the top. The reason we do this is not only so our supervisors know everything we are working on, but also to help us clarify for ourselves our work for the week. Some weeks we have too many hours, so we have to reevaluate our priorities, while other weeks we have extra time to work on upcoming projects or new projects.

Decide how many hours you would like to put toward health counseling this week and make a list of everything you would like to get done, both big and little. Make sure to add in time for phone calls, emails and other miscellaneous tasks. Now identify what the Big Rocks are. What are the items on this list that you absolutely must accomplish this week? And, honestly, how long is it going to take you to make them happen? Be realistic in terms of your time when doing your Big Rocks. Notice if you have a tendency to underestimate or overestimate the amount of time it takes you to do things, and adjust your Big Rocks so that it is an accurate representation of the actual time spent on different projects.

Divide all the work you do into categories, such as Counseling and Preparation, Marketing, Organization and Other. Then list the various projects within each category. For each category, note the amount of hours you plan to spend on this work. You may want to chunk the time down, and list the amount of hours per project.

Doing your Big Rocks every Monday will keep you focused on the important things, and ideally prevent you from spending all your time on the little rocks, or things that don't really matter to you. If you create your Big Rocks each week, realistically representing your time, you will be saved from beating yourself up at the end of the week because you didn't get to the million and one things on your list.

Keep your Big Rocks someplace visible and cross off your tasks as you accomplish them. The next week, list your top five accomplishments at the top of your new Big Rocks to remind yourself how well you are doing. The more you focus on your Big Rocks, and not the little pebbles, the more productive you will be.

The first time you compile your Big Rocks it may take a little while, but after a few weeks, you'll breeze through it in about 20 minutes.

sample big rocks

June 26—June 30 BIG ROCKS

Total Hours = 40

Accomplishments:	signed 1 new client
	attended BNI meeting
	wrote july newsletter
	booked a talk for september
	cleaned office space

COUNSELING & PREPARATION
18 hours

8	client sessions (8)
4	july cooking class
2	prepare for client sessions: review notes, prepare handouts and giveaways
2	stock up on giveaways (books, cds, teas, etc)
2	Health Histories (2)

MARKETING
7 hours

2	lead workshop at community center
2	prepare for workshop: outline, handouts, etc
1	print flyers for workshop
1	contact newspaper about writing an article on summer foods
1	attend weekly BNI meeting

ORGANIZATION
5 hours

file on receipts for tax purposes
update client folders: giveaway checklist and client progress
print Health History forms
create extra new client folders
review finances and budget
follow up with all new contacts

MISC
5 hours

phone
email
travel time

To Do Later This Summer:

workshop at teen camp in august
send press kit to local radio stations
drop in at new spa and talk to manager
send thank-you letters to referral partners
seek out a new chiropractor to be a referral partner
attend weekly BNI meetings
take vacation!

urgent versus important

This exercise is another effective tool to explore where your time goes. There are four quadrants here: important and urgent, not important and urgent, not urgent and important, and not urgent and not important. Everything you do in your life fits into one of these quadrants. Please fill in each quadrant with your regular activities that fit each category.

	Important	Not important
Urgent		
Not urgent		

In which quadrant does most of your time go? Quite frequently, people spend the majority of their time doing things that they categorize as being urgent, but not important, and consequently things that are important get pushed aside. Use this exercise as motivation to cut out anything in your life that is not urgent and not important. Also, cut down the amount of time you spend on things that are urgent, but not important. Put the excess time and energy into things that are important to you, but not urgent.

Excerpted from *The 7 Habits of Highly Effective People: Powerful Lessons in Personal Change* by Stephen R. Covey, Fireside, $15.00.

furthering your education

As a student at Integrative Nutrition, you already know enough to be a health counselor and to have a positive effect on anyone who comes your way. You do not need to know every little detail about nutrition and health in order to help your clients. With that said, furthering your education beyond what you learn with us can be exciting and energizing. Through reading books and attending classes, workshops or retreats on topics related to health, you can re-inspire yourself about your career.

Make a list of topics that are related to your work as a health counselor and that you would like to learn more about:

1. _____

2. _____

3. _____

4. _____

5. _____

How much money can you allocate in the next six months towards furthering your education?

_____

(Even if it's zero, you can still learn almost anything. You can barter with a teacher, attend free seminars or borrow books from the library.)

Places such as The Open Center in New York City, Omega in Rhinebeck, New York and Texas, and Esalen and Heartwood, both in California, offer weekend, weeklong and month-long classes on topics related to health and wellness. Check them out, along with any other resources in your area. What are some classes, workshops or books that are within your budget and related to your areas of interest?

1. _____

2. _____

3. _____

4. _____

5. _____

A gentle warning about getting addicted to workshops and brain candy: you already know so much more than the average person. Your listening skills and natural intelligence are what makes you a powerful health counselor, not how many books you've read or degrees you have. Further your education for fun and for your own interest, not because you think you don't know enough.

need motivation?

If you lack motivation, look inside and be honest with yourself about what you are experiencing. Why have you not been prioritizing health counseling? Only you know the answer to that question. If you aren't sure, journal about what you are going through and get feedback from your mentor, buddy and other support people.

In our experience, lack of motivation is often caused by fear of success or failure. Deep down you want to be a health counselor, but you lack confidence for one reason or another. You probably have thought patterns from a long time ago that still go on in your head and say that you aren't good enough or smart enough to do what your heart desires.

A helpful analogy here is the Hudson River. Everyone thinks it flows one way, downstream into the ocean. But the river is very deep and influenced by tides. Although it's hard to tell on the surface, the river's flow actually changes direction several times a day, sending water back upstream. This is similar to what happens inside of you when you say you want something, but underneath it all you are too afraid. Powerful feelings can pull you in the opposite direction from where you really want to go. Take a moment to think about any fears you have around being a health counselor. Don't be shy. Everyone has them. It's totally normal.

common fears students face
- I'm not healthy enough, so who am I to be telling other people what to eat and how to exercise?
- If I actually succeed at this, then I'll have to be perfect all the time.
- If I work for myself, I'll always be thinking about work.
- If I make money, I'll have to support everyone else in my family.
- If I outgrow my old lifestyle, I'll lose all my friends.
- It's not safe to depend on myself for a paycheck. I could go broke.
- If I do what I want instead of what my parents want, they won't love me anymore.
- What if my clients don't get well? They might blame me and be angry.
- If I own a business, I will lose free time and flexibility.
- I'm not smart enough to make good decisions, so my business could fail.
- If I spend all day listening to people talk about their problems, I'll feel depressed.
- If I get up in front of people and talk about nutrition, people will laugh at me.
- If I'm always helping other people, no one will help me.
- If I change careers, I will lose credibility with my business associates.
- If I do what I want to do, everyone will think I'm selfish.

Make a list of potential reasons why you might not want to be a health counselor.

1. _____

2. _____

3. _____

4. _____

5. _____

6. _____

7. _____

8. _____

9. _____

10. _____

It is worthwhile to spend some time acknowledging your fears. See if you can decipher where these fears originated. Remember that the past is over and anything is possible in the present. Use your counselor, a journal and the support at the school to work through your fear, procrastination and self-doubt.

On occasion, people simply are not motivated to be health counselors because it is not their calling in life. They may come to the school and start out as health counselors, but end up deciding that becoming a full-time mom is where their true happiness lies, or that their lifelong dream was to move to another country. Whatever your dreams are, we want them to come true for you. Know that even if you don't have clients in a six-month program, you will always be a source of inspiration and health to those who know you.

career future-building

What would you like to accomplish in your career by the end of the week?

_____

_____

_____

_____

What would you like to accomplish in your career by the end of the month?

_____

_____

_____

_____

_____

What would you like to accomplish in your career by the end of the year?

_____

_____

_____

_____

2 years?

_____

_____

_____

_____

5 years?

_____

_____

_____

_____

10 years?

_____

_____

_____

_____

20 years?

_____

_____

_____

_____

Beyond:

_____

_____

_____

_____

_____

The principal motivating factor in life is goals. If you do not have them, you won't know what you are working towards. Regardless of where your passions lie—either in health counseling or another career—setting goals for your future provides motivation. Then you must do the work to turn these dreams into your reality.

you create your future

There is a direct correlation between your thoughts and the future you create for yourself. The more confidently you move forward with your business, the more victory will come to you. Whatever your goals are, act as if you have already accomplished them. Carry yourself as if you have the number of clients you want. Talk to potential clients as if you know they are going to sign up for your program and that it is going to be one of the best things that ever happened to them. Every time you catch yourself thinking that this might not work out, change your thought to something more positive.

When an opportunity to expand your business comes your way, jump on it! Don't let potential clients, referral partners or leads get by you. Trust your instincts when it comes to people. And when your gut tells you that there is an opportunity coming your way, take it and then give gratitude. Gratitude is a way of thanking the universe and inviting more opportunities.

List three things you feel confident and positive about right now.

1. _____

2. _____

3. _____

focus on opportunities, not obstacles

Successful people focus on opportunities, not obstacles. They see potential growth, not potential loss.

It comes down to the age-old question, "Is the glass half empty or half full?" We're not talking about positive thinking here; we're talking about your habitual perspective on the world. You don't want to make choices out of fear, to constantly be scanning for what could go wrong in any situation.

Successful people expect to succeed. Try to be optimistic. Act upon the mindset, "It will work because I'll make it work." Have confidence in your abilities, have confidence in your creativity, and believe that, should the doo-doo hit the fan, you can find another way to succeed.

If you want to experience success, focus on the opportunities in everything. If you focus on opportunities, opportunities will abound for you. If you focus on obstacles, obstacles abound for you. It's simple. Your field of focus determines what you find in life.

Take this as your motto: action beats inaction. Successful people get started. They trust that once they get in the game, they can make intelligent decisions in the present moment, make corrections and adjust their sales along the way.

Adapted from *Secrets of the Millionaire Mind: Mastering the Inner Game of Wealth* by T. Harv Eker, Harper Business, $19.95.

reflecting on your accomplishments

Building your health counseling business is a journey, not a destination. It is not a problem that has to be solved; it is a process through which you will learn what being successful means and looks like to you. If you can develop the habit of recognizing your accomplishments along this journey, you will have the added bonus of experiencing joy. When you stop to recognize how well you are doing, you put focus on your own prosperity and invite in even more. One way to appreciate your progress is to take an inventory before bed each night, and appreciate everything you did well that day. Another way is to post your to-do list or Big Rocks somewhere in your office, and when you have accomplished something, check it off the list. This is incredibly satisfying. By doing this you will see exactly how much you have done. Consistently remind yourself that you are an amazing person, and you are doing the best that you can.

What are you most proud of regarding your health counseling business?

_____

_____

_____

_____

What has been your greatest accomplishment in the past six months?

_____

_____

_____

_____

What obstacles have you overcome to be where you are today?

_____

_____

_____

_____

_____

What concrete benefits have you brought to your clients, friends and family, and to yourself, as a result of committing to health counseling?

_____

_____

_____

_____

List 10 things you love about yourself.

1. _____

2. _____

3. _____

4. _____

5. _____

6. _____

7. _____

8. _____

9. _____

10. _____

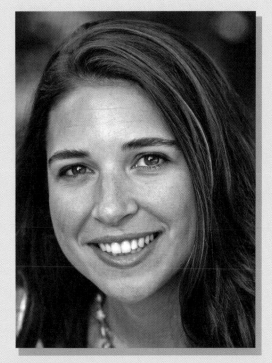

Lisa Graham
New York, NY
lgrahamiin@yahoo.com
2004 Graduate

Growing up, I was involved with exercise and sports, but I never paid attention to what I was eating. When I was diagnosed with optic neuritis, which is associated with multiple sclerosis, I realized that my poor eating habits were affecting my health. I was eager to learn as much nutrition information as possible, so when I came across the Integrative Nutrition catalog, it sounded perfect for me.

At the school, I became clear about my passions and where I wanted to go with my career. I know what it's like to be scared around my health and to feel there is nowhere to turn when doctors are not helpful. As a health counselor, I support people in the process of exploring alternative routes, listening to their body's signals, and using food to restore their health and vitality.

I work fulltime as an executive assistant in a real estate development company and run my health counseling business parttime during evenings and weekends. My clients are primarily busy professionals who are looking to eat healthier, lose weight and use nutrition to prevent disease.

I am always thinking of new ideas and ways to network. I affiliated with a spa and work there one evening a week as a health counselor. I also recently blended image consulting into my practice. I have a college degree in fashion, and it is one of my passions. Everyone has an individual personal style and I love helping people find what it is. I give them tools to work with their body type and portray an image that is in line with their goals. It is a natural extension of health counseling, and it blends into my business beautifully.

Getting clear around money and my worth as a health counselor was a crucial part of my process. Originally, I charged $100 per month and I steadily increased my price to $300 per month. I am confident about my program and feel comfortable charging this rate. My guidance and support are worth it. It feels good to do what I love and get paid well for it.

It is really beneficial to deal with money at the first session and get payment for the entire program up-front, whether in one lump sum or post-dated checks. It gets too confusing and inconvenient if I don't take care of it at the beginning. If I'm going to work with someone, I need them to be 100% committed. Paying up-front keeps my clients focused and dedicated to the program.

I love health counseling because I can support people and see their lives change for the better. Minor changes make huge differences, and giving a little knowledge goes a long way. I continue to learn and improve myself as I teach my clients to learn and improve themselves. Anything is possible if you put your mind to it and take consistent action.

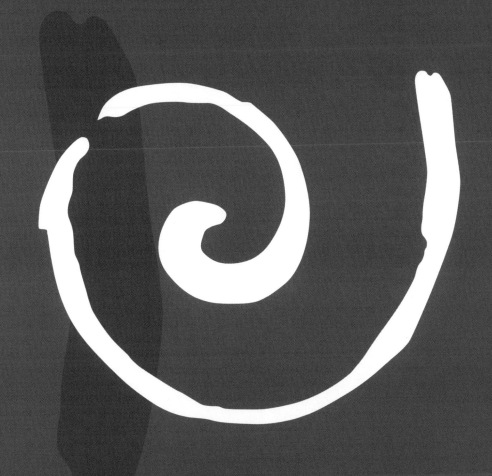

chapter ten

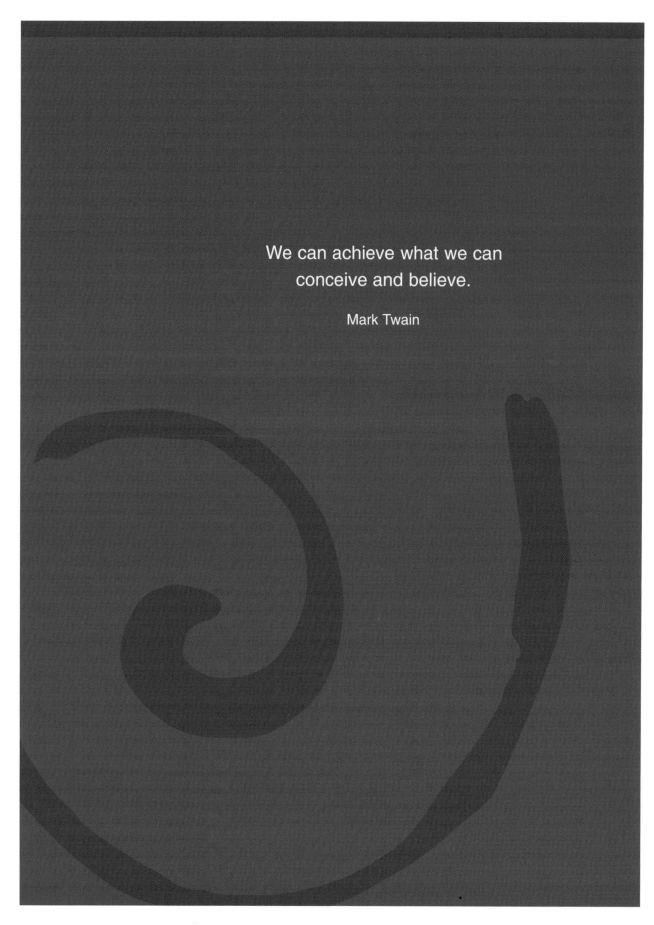

We can achieve what we can
conceive and believe.

Mark Twain

as you near the end of the Professional Training Program, you are probably making some decisions about where to take your health counseling practice. Will this be a part-time adventure, to make supplemental income on top of your current career? Will you use health counseling only with your family and community without earning money from it? Or will you make health counseling your full-time career that provides income and fulfillment for years to come? This chapter has helpful information no matter where you are with health counseling, but it focuses on how to develop the skills you need to be a long-term, full-time health counselor.

business owner mentality

It is a high priority for us to have our alumni experience tremendous success with health counseling long after graduation. After all, the way we are going to change the healthcare system in America is by having our graduates work with as many people as possible.

If you enjoy helping clients, and can see yourself doing this work full time, you will eventually have to shift from having a private practice, with one to 15 clients at a time, to being a business owner. The difference is this: people with a private practice focus on the few clients they have, do marketing and networking to maintain a number of clients they enjoy, and invest minimally in business growth. By becoming a business owner, you are saying to yourself and the world, "This is what I want to do with my life." You make health counseling your career and commit to doing this work for an extended period of time. You work to grow, enhance and stabilize your business over the long term.

One way to measure if you are ready to make the leap into a full-time career as a health counselor is by looking at your finances. Have you been able to easily pay your bills over the past six months with the money you've made from health counseling? If so, you are definitely ready to move forward, knowing it's only going to get better from here. If you haven't been able to pay your bills easily, it's probably best to focus on getting more clients before jumping into heavy-duty business building.

keys to achievement

- focus—Stay focused on your goals. Use the time management tools to ensure that you are using your time to work towards your top priorities.

- evidence—Evaluate how you are doing. Be honest with yourself. Are you working too hard or not hard enough? Have you accomplished enough this week, and are you able to take a day off without guilt? Or have you been slacking and need to up the ante? Constantly measure your level of effort and compare it to your results. This will help you refine your tactics and make smarter decisions.

- direction—Complete your Big Rocks, and include scheduling workshops, networking events and marketing steps each week. If you complete everything on your Big Rocks, you will see results.

- motivation—Set up reward systems for yourself. Try not to have these involve food. Maybe you get a massage with every new client you sign, or if you reach your target for new clients at the end of the month, you buy yourself a new outfit. Also, remind yourself about why you are doing this work, and have goals ahead to keep you working towards something in the future.

- accountability—Have someone other than yourself in your life who will ask you what you've done so far and what's next. Be accountable to this person. They could be your buddy, your counselor or your board of directors.

- perspective – Get a different point of view on your progress or challenges. Just hearing your problem restated by another person can give you insight that might help you find a solution. When you are feeling low, it's also great to have someone as your personal cheerleader.

- support—No matter where you are in your business development, having a mentor and a support team is essential to your success. You may use friends, spouses or family members for this purpose, but if you are determined to do this work fulltime, having a business coach is extremely beneficial. There are many experienced graduates available to help you navigate through your journey. Our graduate directory and Case Histories book are great resources for finding successful graduates

- prioritize—A lot of opportunities will come your way as a health counselor. Stay focused on what you want to achieve, and prioritize the things that will help you reach your goals more quickly. A rule of thumb employed by many successful graduates is to prioritize the things that bring in clients!

- enjoy yourself—Whenever things get stressful or dull, remember that you are the boss of you, and you can reinvent yourself and your business. Add fun activities to your routine. Take a class on something you always wanted to learn. Try a new food or recipe and then share it with your clients. This work never has to be monotonous. And, at the end of each day, appreciate yourself for your efforts and for doing your best.

adapted from *Get Clients Now!* by CJ Hayden

Taking on the mentality of a business owner can actually decrease stress. This may seem counter-intuitive, but think about it. Everyone knows all businesses take a few years to build. You can approach your business slowly and methodically. The ebbs and flows of your business growth should be expected. Every corporation and business expert knows that you can't implement all your ideas for change at once. They strategize the best moves to make, measure the success of those moves and then decide the next move.

Approach your health counseling business in the same way. Once you decide to pursue this work fulltime, pick one area you want to focus on. Keep on track with this single point of focus. For example, you may want to increase your visibility, so you book workshops and beef up your PR. Do this for a month or two and measure your results. Is your phone ringing more often? Do you have more Health Histories this month? What worked and what didn't work? Once you evaluate this strategy, decide your next move. Always keep in mind that your business is a constant work in progress. You don't have to do it all at once.

raising your rates

Graduation is a perfect time to raise your rates. You can raise them by a little or by a lot, depending on your comfort level and what you are already charging.

Remember when you were little and learning to ride a bike? First you rode with training wheels. You thought you needed them, but eventually your mom or dad took the wheels off. When you rode without them for the first time you probably realized that you could have taken them off much sooner. Your body already knew how to balance perfectly on the bike. It was your mind that needed longer to develop confidence. Raising your rates is like taking off your training wheels. It's like saying to yourself and the world, "I can do it!"

It's time to take the training wheels off your business. Your program is priceless and has been from the first time you sat down with a client. But you needed time to develop confidence. Now you are ready to openly own your own value and charge what you are worth.

In our experience $250 per month is a good amount to charge as a newly graduated health counselor. Maybe you are comfortable with charging more or less than that. Wherever you are is okay, but be careful not to undersell yourself. Many students and graduates have shared that when they charged $150 per month it was harder to get clients than when they increased their rates to $250. This is because $250 per month is a better indicator of the true value of the program. When people hear that it costs that much, they understand that it must really be valuable.

What do you charge for your program now? _____

What services do your clients get for that cost?

_____

_____

_____

List results your clients have received from working with you so far. List benefits your friends and family get simply by having your presence in their lives. What would you pay a professional for these benefits and results?

_____

_____

_____

_____

_____

List everything that has gone into making you the invaluable counselor you are today. Include natural talents, unique skills, career experience, travel, personal growth and development, books read, workshops attended, formal education and anything else in your life. How much would you pay a professional with this level of experience to be your support person?

_____

_____

_____

_____

_____

If you asked your biggest fan how much you should charge for your program, what would they say?

_____

_____

What will be the new cost of your program when you graduate?

_____

_____

setting financial goals

As a business owner, you no longer have a boss setting your salary. You get to decide how much money you want or need to make, and then make it happen. Your financial plan helps you determine how many clients you need to see at a given time, which helps you organize your marketing plan. Financial planning can be fun and empowering as you learn to take charge of your money in a new way.

List your monthly personal expenses:

rent/mortgage: $_____

food: $_____

clothing: $_____

entertainment: $_____

health insurance: $_____

self-care: $_____

other household expenses: $_____

$_____

$_____

$_____

$_____

$_____

$_____

List your monthly business expenses:

phones: $_____

internet: $_____

office supplies: $_____

client giveaways: $_____

cooking class materials: $_____

other event expenses: $_____

taxes: $_____

other: $_____

$_____

$_____

$_____

$_____

$_____

$_____

How much would you like to save or invest per month? $_____

Add up all these expenses. This how much you want to make per month: $ _____

Multiply by 12. This is your desired yearly income: $ _____

How much will come from your health counseling business? $ _____

How much will come from other ventures? $ _____

How many clients will you need?

1. List the amount that will come from counseling each month: $ _____

2. List your monthly program fee: $ _____

3. Divide line 1 by line 2: _____

This is the number of clients you need to see each month in order to reach your desired income. For example, if you want to make $6,500 from health counseling this month, and you charge $295 per month, you will need to see 22 clients this month to make the income you desire. Revisit your marketing strategy to see how it can help you to meet your goal in an efficient, effective way.

health insurance

As a self-employed person, you will have to purchase health insurance yourself if you need it. Most health insurance options for small businesses and sole proprietors are expensive, but as today's work-force becomes more mobile and flexible, new options are being created all the time. Plans often vary by state, so research options in your area and keep an eye out for any new plans that might offer you a better deal.

individual plans with major insurers

You don't need to be employed by a big company to be covered by popular providers like Blue Cross Blue Shield, HIP, Aetna and others. You can buy an individual plan directly from the company. HMO options are usually the most affordable, ranging from about $300 to $500 a month. In general, the higher your deductible, the lower your monthly premium and vice versa. Visit each company website to get specific prices for plans.

plans for freelancers and sole proprietors

Because many self-employed people cannot afford to buy their insurance from the big companies, cities or professional groups sometimes pool their resources to offer basic plans at more affordable rates. For example, in the New York City area you can purchase insurance through Working Today's Freelancers Union (www.workingtoday.org), Brooklyn HealthWorks (www.brooklynhealthworks.com) and Healthy New York (www.healthyny.com). Monthly premiums for an individual run between $200 and $300. You can also buy coverage for family members.

coverage through another employer

If you have a spouse or close relative with a good insurance plan at their job, you can be covered on their plan. This could cost the same or more as paying for your own basic insurance, but you might get more benefits or more flexible options. Also, if you are health counseling part time and working somewhere else part time, your employer may be able to cover your health insurance needs.

hiring help

To run a thriving business, you are going to need support. Help can come from your family, friends and support team. It should also come from paid professionals. It is worth it to invest in yourself so that you can have a great life and get your agenda accomplished. Your paid employees and support people are there to help you do just that.

when to hire an assistant

If you have a solid practice and are consistently making $75 to $100 per hour, you can hire an assistant. This person will take care of basic tasks, like typing and filing, for $12 to $15 per hour, leaving you much more time to market your business and sign clients. Most likely you will not need your assistant to work full time. You can set up hours that work best for you. They could come in one full day each week or for a few hours each day. Delegate tasks that take time away from signing clients and that you don't need to do in person. Depending on your needs, your assistant could organize your papers, order supplies, book appointments, buy your groceries or research new places for you to give workshops.

hiring additional health counselors

Signing up too many clients is a good problem to have. If you want to keep a high number of clients in your business, but you can't handle seeing all of them, hire another health counselor. Here's how this can work. Do Health Histories and close deals with clients, letting them know that you will assign them to a counselor in your business that best suits their needs. Then pay another counselor to work with some clients. Negotiate an agreement with your counselor about how much they will be paid. Will you pay them hourly? Split the client fee 50/50? 40/60? It's totally up to you.

If and when you hire other counselors, you may want to incorporate education into their benefits. You can take them to time management or personal growth and development conferences to help them improve their counseling and business skills. You can also provide self-care benefits like organic meals in the office, weekly yoga classes or monthly massages. Having other counselors in your business can be very rewarding. Your team can have lunch together, discuss client health concerns, share laughs and disappointments and generally support one another.

hiring other professionals

What are other areas of your life where you could you save time, money and energy by paying someone to help you? For example, is it worth it to spend five hours cleaning your home this week? Or could you use that time to sign more clients and pay someone $100 to clean your house? Is it worth it to spend extra time commuting across town for your yoga class? Or could you hire a yoga instructor to come right to your door?

Professionals you could hire include:
- accountant
- bookkeeper
- business coach

- cook
- cleaning person
- massage therapist
- private yoga instructor
- writer or writing coach

If you are a new business owner, you might feel uncomfortable being "the boss" and paying others to do what you ask. Actually this is a great way to practice knowing your own worth and being "on top of the food chain." Recognize that you are up to something exciting that others will want to be a part of. Many people would love to work for a passionate, committed business owner who runs their business with love and integrity and who is making the world a better place. Over time you will figure out a management style that works best for you. Build your confidence by leading your team and noticing that other people are happy to support you.

giving back

Chances are your life is pretty good. You may only see what is not working for you. In reality, many people in the world are hungry, sick, poor and live without a home or a family. When you realize how others are living and compare it to how you are living, you'll see that most people in the world would love to have your life.

We encourage you to find ways to give freely to those who have less than you. In your local community there may be senior citizens, children, people with illnesses or underprivileged families who would benefit greatly from your services and cannot afford them. Sharing your expertise with those less fortunate can be hugely rewarding for you, and they will benefit from access to priceless information they would not have if not for your services. Here a few ways you can give back:

- Work with a school to offer an inexpensive group program to teens.
- Donate free sessions, cooking classes or workshops to a benefit auction.
- Organize a group of volunteers to cook a healthy meal for a soup kitchen.
- Work with a YMCA or community center to offer a group program for free or at reduced rates.
- Ask your local church, school or retirement home if they would like you to give a free talk about wellness.

You can also give to community organizations that are working on important health issues. Grassroots organizations are often volunteer-run and under-funded. They could benefit greatly from your time, expertise or financial donation. Some movements you could support include:

- advocating for clean air and water
- protecting the quality of organic foods
- raising public awareness about the dangers of sugar and junk foods
- fighting the influence of the food industry on the government and media

ways to expand your health counseling career

- Run retreats.
- Write a book.
- Get a radio show
- Get a cooking show.
- Own a wellness center.
- Create your own magazine.
- Work in a hospital or doctor's office.
- Be a corporate wellness consultant.
- Be a school food expert or activist.
- Get a column in a newspaper or magazine.

school food

One area that many of our graduates are involved with is school food. Today people are more aware than ever that sugar, junk and low-quality foods are hurting our children. Parents and community groups are starting to press for more nutritious foods in schools so that our children can be healthy and have a great future.

In spring 2006 the government ruled that sugary soft drinks could no longer be sold in elementary and middle schools. By summer 2006 all schools nationwide had to have wellness policies. These are important steps forward, but there is a lot more to do. Schools and parent groups need active support to learn what foods are healthy for their children and how to get those foods into school cafeterias.

How you can help:
- Offer free wellness workshops directly to kids.
- Drop by your local school at lunchtime and see what the kids are being fed.
- Ask the head of the PTA what is already being done to improve school food.
- Offer free wellness workshops to PTA members, school administrators or concerned parents.
- Find out what your state and local government says about school food and organize a letter-writing campaign.

Other resources for supporting the healthy school food movement:
- www.ecoliteracy.org/programs/index.html
- www.healthyschoollunches.org (for New York State)
- www.angrymoms.org (by Integrative Nutrition graduates)

Giving generously to people and organizations that need support can be an important part of fulfilling your vision. The more you understand that the universe supports you to achieve your dreams and to always have enough, the easier it is to share your time, energy and expertise with others.

your vision

You are ultimately in charge of your business and the direction you'd like to go.
The clearer your intentions and vision for your practice become, the more likely it is that you will
be successful. Your vision, or mission, is simply that which you'd like to accomplish in your business.
It is the compass for your business, and gives you direction on how to move forward with purpose
and clarity. This vision will keep you going every day, even when things aren't going so well or
according to your plan.

It is important to consider why you do this work and your higher goals for your business.
Explore the difference you want to make with this work and what influence you want to have on
your clients.

Why do I do this work?

_____

_____

_____

_____

What motivates me?

_____

_____

_____

_____

Who do I really want to help?

_____

_____

_____

_____

What difference do I want to make in the world?

_____

_____

_____

_____

_____

_____

When am I inspired?

_____

_____

_____

_____

_____

_____

What is my life purpose?

_____

_____

_____

_____

_____

_____

macro-vision

It's helpful to break your vision down into a macro-vision and a micro-vision. A macro-vision is similar to a mission statement. It is the ultimate goal of your business and maybe even your life. Your macro-vision drives all the choices you make. It answers the questions of why you were born and what impact you want to have on the world. Your macro-vision is bigger than you are.

Here's an example: The macro-vision of the Institute for Integrative Nutrition is to transform the healthcare system in America and throughout the world, and by doing so to make the world a happier, healthier place.

Take a moment now to write out the macro-vision of your business. Use the vision exercise above and the mission statement exercise from Chapter 4 to help you.

_____

_____

_____

_____

_____

_____

_____

_____

_____

Now refine your macro-vision. See if you can express it in just two or three sentences.

_____

_____

_____

_____

_____

_____

micro-vision

Your micro-vision is what you will focus on in the coming months to make your macro-vision a reality. It answers the question of what you are going to do today to support your macro-vision. For example, if your macro-vision is to improve the quality of life for children in your community, your micro-vision may be to get involved in local schools and create a plan to upgrade school lunches.

As a health counselor, many projects and opportunities will come your way. Your micro-vision helps you make the day-to-day choices about what to get involved in. Guage each opportunity that comes your way and only take on projects that are a match for you. Know that it is okay to turn down opportunities if they are not in alignment with your vision. In some cases you may be offered projects that are in line with your macro-vision, but not your current micro-vision. It is okay to postpone those projects until a later date.

Your macro-vision will stay more or less constant throughout your life and practice. Your micro-vision will shift every few months as you complete projects, expand your horizons and discover new ways to meet your goals. Revisit your micro-vision often to make sure it is still relevant and helping you to fulfill your overall vision.

Write down your micro-vision for your business in the next six months.

_____

_____

_____

_____

_____

_____

_____

_____

_____

_____

_____

lifelong learning

One of the best ways to build and maintain your business is to stay connected to the Integrative Nutrition community. You will have access to educational tools and programs designed especially for graduates, including conferences, alumni OEFs, alumni Local Study Chapters, the alumni newsletter and teleclasses. We are always upgrading our services for alumni so that they can stay up to date on cutting-edge nutrition news and business-building techniques.

If you are looking for immediate, immeasurable levels of support to propel your business forward, you can apply for the Immersion Program. Most graduates who attend do so right after their PTP year to maintain their momentum. Immersion is the best way to upgrade your business right out of the gate. You will quickly gain counseling experience, while learning the next level of business skills and receiving support from some of our most successful graduates.

Integrative Nutrition is a community of people working together to effect great change in the world. We strongly recommend you surround yourself with other graduates. Your health counselor friends are invaluable. They will be able to listen to you and offer you the business and personal advice that only other health counselors can give. Please stay connected to the people and resources you need to continue to learn and grow.

we appreciate you

We know that you had to overcome a lot to make it to Integrative Nutrition. For many of you it has meant reprioritizing your life, traveling long distances or letting go of personal fears and limitations. We truly appreciate you for dedicating yourself to making this world a happier, healthier place to live.

Thank you for all the hard work you put into being a student. Thank you for being a part of our community. We are proud to have you as a graduate of our school and hope you will stay connected and continue to work with us to make our vision a reality. We wish you a happy, healthy future, filled with great success.

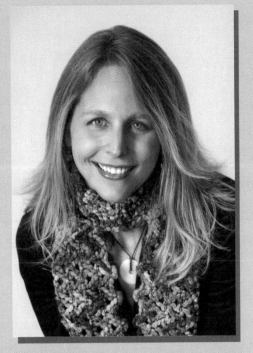

Robin Peglow
Denver, CO
robin@signsoflifehealth.com
2000 Graduate

I used to be a staff recruiter for a summer camp in upstate New York. I wasn't making the kind of impact I wanted to be making in the world; I knew I wanted to live a bigger life. When I first heard about Integrative Nutrition, I wasn't sure if I wanted to go, but the more I thought about it, the more I realized that health counseling was the perfect career for me.

My year at Integrative Nutrition was the best year of my life. It was great to be part of a community that was really up to something. The school taught me to honor myself, dream big and choose my own life. It had been my dream to live in Colorado, and after graduation I moved out here.

My health counseling practice focuses on supporting women to discover their "soul food," that which nourishes inspiration, intuition and rebalances the feminine within strength. Most of my clients are women who are generally happy in their lives, yet have a subtle sense that there is something more, a deeper experience available to them that they're not sure how to find. They're often motivated career women and moms who've hit a sticky spot of "Now what?" My program is a formula for helping these women access their wisdom and intuition, so they can begin living the kind of life they desire, one that will make them truly happy.

I have created a series of classes called Access Your Power Within™ that support women in aligning with their goals, values, intuitions and inspirations. In just over three years I have led 70 women through this program, and it's great to see the difference it has made in their lives. Based on this work, I wrote, and now sell *Power On Purpose: A Daily Guide to Living in Your Power,* a self-care guide and companion book.

I used to call myself the best-kept secret in Denver, but that's no longer true. I knew only two people when I arrived here, and I built my business from scratch. Since then, I've been interviewed for the TV news and published in several magazines, reaching well over 30,000 subscribers. My network of supporters and referral partners has grown large. And now I'm positioning myself to support even more people by running retreats and expanding my publications.

One of the challenges of building a practice is that we often don't know exactly how it's going to be or what to expect. Learn to let go of your fear and be graceful in the face of uncertainty. Be willing to let things evolve. We often want it to happen right now, but many lessons must come slowly. It takes time to lay the foundation.

I do this work because it energizes me, and because I love supporting people to get inspired. I am fostering relationships in my workshops and creating a more conscious community in Denver. My business is going incredibly well and totally expresses who I am. I'm so grateful, and I can't imagine doing anything else.

index